Diabetic smoothie cookbook 2024

Balancing Blood Sugar: Delectable Blends for Health-Conscious Diabetics

Ennis James

Table of Contents

Introduction

In the quaint suburban town of Willowbrook, nestled between
vibrant gardens and bustling community centers, lived
58-year-old Martha Rivers, a retired school teacher with a newly
discovered passion for health and wellness. Diagnosed with type 2
diabetes three years ago, Martha had initially felt overwhelmed.
The countless food restrictions and the daunting task of
managing her blood sugar levels seemed almost insurmountable.
But her indomitable spirit led her to a breakthrough discovery:
"Diabetic Smoothie Cookbook 2024," a guide that promised not
just recipes, but a new approach to life.

One sunny morning, while sipping a green apple spinach
smoothie from her porch, Martha reflected on her journey. Before
discovering the cookbook, breakfast had been a predictable affair
of bland oatmeal or a plain piece of toast. Now, her mornings
were invigorated with smoothies like the Berry Oat Breakfast and
the Cinnamon Roll Smoothie, each recipe meticulously crafted to
fit her diabetic dietary needs without sacrificing flavor.

The guide was more than just a collection of recipes; it was a
fountain of knowledge. With sections dedicated to understanding
diabetes and the nutritional impact of ingredients, Martha learned
to tailor her diet to her body's needs. The book emphasized low
glycemic index fruits, healthy fats, and fibers that helped maintain
her blood sugar levels, all while allowing her to enjoy rich, savory

blends like the Tomato Basil or the Cucumber Mint Refresh at lunch.

Her afternoons were now punctuated with preparations of dinner smoothies, which transformed her view on what dinner could look like. The Sweet Potato and Cinnamon Smoothie became a comforting favorite during the chilly autumn evenings, and the Creamy Avocado Cacao was a guilt-free treat that even her grandchildren begged for during their visits.

Word of Martha's newfound vitality and the colorful smoothies she carried everywhere spread through Willowbrook. Her friends, curious and eager, gathered at her home for a tasting event where Martha showcased her favorite recipes from the guide. Each sip their friends took was met with surprised delight and genuine interest.

"I never knew managing diabetes could be this delicious and simple!" exclaimed Linda, one of her closest friends, as she savored the Kale and Green Apple Smoothie. The gathering turned into an impromptu Q&A session, where Martha explained how the cookbook had taught her about the effects of different foods on blood sugar levels, the importance of fiber, and how to indulge wisely.

Inspired by her transformation, Martha started a blog, "Martha's Smoothie Corner," where she shared her daily smoothie creations, tips for managing diabetes, and snippets of her life in Willowbrook. The response was overwhelmingly positive, with readers from across the country writing to thank her for making their journey with diabetes less daunting and more enjoyable.

"Diabetic Smoothie Cookbook 2024" was more than just a book; it was a companion that had guided Martha towards a healthier, more joyful lifestyle. It promised and delivered a simple, sustainable way to manage diabetes through delicious, nutritious smoothies, bringing color and sweetness back into her life without compromising her health.

For anyone sitting on the fence about purchasing the cookbook, Martha had one message: "This isn't just about recipes; it's about reclaiming your health and joy in eating. It's one of the best investments you could make for your health, happiness, and taste buds!"

And so, the Diabetic Smoothie Cookbook 2024 became not just a bestseller but a beacon of hope for many, guided by Martha's enthusiastic endorsement and heartfelt story.

Understanding Diabetes

Diabetes is a metabolic disorder that impairs the body's ability to process blood glucose, commonly known as blood sugar. In healthy individuals, the pancreas produces insulin, a hormone that facilitates the movement of sugar from the bloodstream into the cells, where it's used for energy. However, in people with diabetes, this process is disrupted due to inadequate insulin production or the body's inability to use insulin effectively, leading to elevated blood sugar levels. Chronic high blood sugar can lead to serious health complications, including heart disease, kidney damage, and nerve dysfunction.

Type 1 diabetes is an autoimmune condition where the body's immune system attacks the insulin-producing cells in the pancreas. This type often manifests early in life and requires daily insulin injections for management. Type 2 diabetes, which is more common, typically develops in adults and is largely influenced by lifestyle factors such as diet and physical activity. It can often be managed or even reversed with dietary changes, exercise, and weight loss, alongside medication.

Managing diabetes effectively requires maintaining a balanced diet that stabilizes blood sugar levels and prevents fluctuations. Smoothies, as part of this diet, offer a unique advantage. They can be tailored to include fiber-rich vegetables and fruits, protein, and healthy fats, which all help to slow down the absorption of glucose, thereby preventing spikes in blood sugar levels. The right blend of ingredients can create a nutritious meal that satisfies dietary needs without compromising taste or nutrition.

The Diabetic Smoothie Cookbook 2024 is designed to simplify this aspect of dietary management for those living with diabetes. Each recipe in the cookbook provides a balanced mix of nutrients that cater specifically to the needs of diabetics, focusing on low glycemic index fruits and vegetables, fibers, and proteins that support blood sugar control. The inclusion of specific nutrients in these smoothies can also aid in overall health, supporting cardiovascular health, digestion, and energy levels.

Moreover, the convenience of smoothies makes them an excellent choice for individuals with a busy lifestyle. Preparing a nutritious smoothie can be a quick process, and for many diabetics, this ease of preparation ensures they do not skip meals, which is crucial for preventing low blood sugar levels. Additionally, smoothies can be consumed on the go, making them a practical solution for maintaining a healthy diet even during busy days.

Education about ingredient selection is crucial for diabetics. The cookbook educates readers on choosing ingredients that add flavor without excess sugar, such as using spices like cinnamon or nutmeg, which can also have blood sugar-lowering effects. Understanding the impact of each ingredient allows individuals to customize their smoothie recipes further to suit their taste preferences and nutritional requirements.

In essence, the Diabetic Smoothie Cookbook 2024 serves as a practical tool in the dietary management of diabetes, offering delicious, easy-to-make recipes that are aligned with a diabetic's health requirements. The smoothies featured in the cookbook are more than just meals; they are part of a broader approach to health that empowers individuals with diabetes to manage their condition proactively and enjoyably, integrating wholesome nutrition into their daily routine without feeling restricted.

Benefits of Smoothies for Diabetics

Smoothies can be an excellent dietary addition for individuals managing diabetes, providing a way to consume a wide array of essential nutrients effortlessly. They allow for the integration of low glycemic index fruits, vegetables, and proteins into a diabetic's diet, helping to maintain stable blood sugar levels. Carefully selected ingredients can minimize spikes in glucose, making smoothies particularly beneficial for glucose control. By blending ingredients like berries, spinach, and protein powders, individuals can create a meal that is both nutrient-rich and blood sugar friendly.

The versatility of smoothies is especially valuable for those with diabetes. With the ability to adjust ingredients according to nutritional needs and personal taste preferences, smoothies never become monotonous. They can be tailored to include fiber-rich greens and fruits, healthy fats from avocados or nuts, and proteins such as Greek yogurt or silken tofu. This makes it easier for diabetics to manage their diet without feeling restricted, as they can enjoy a variety of flavors and textures while still adhering to a health-conscious eating plan.

Smoothies are also an effective way to manage portion control, a crucial element in diabetic diet management. By preparing smoothies at home, individuals can precisely measure their ingredients, ensuring they consume the right amount of carbohydrates, proteins, and fats. This control helps prevent overeating and makes it easier to calculate insulin needs for those who are insulin dependent.

The inclusion of high-fiber ingredients in smoothies is another significant benefit. Fiber slows the absorption of sugar into the bloodstream, which helps prevent rapid spikes in blood glucose levels. Ingredients like chia seeds, flaxseeds, or oats can be ground and added to smoothies to enhance their fiber content without significantly altering the taste. These additions help promote a feeling of fullness, reducing the urge to snack between meals, which is beneficial for weight management.

For diabetics, consuming adequate amounts of vegetables and fruits can sometimes be challenging. Smoothies provide a convenient and appealing way to increase intake of these essential food groups. The natural sweetness of fruits can help satisfy sugar cravings in a healthy way, while the inclusion of vegetables increases the nutritional value of the smoothie without adding excessive calories or carbohydrates.

Smoothies also offer hydrating benefits, as many fruits and vegetables are high in water content. Hydration is particularly important for diabetics as it helps regulate blood sugar levels and supports kidney function. Additionally, the ease of preparation and the portability of smoothies make them an excellent option for busy individuals who might otherwise skip meals or resort to less healthy options when on the go.

Lastly, the antioxidant properties of many smoothie ingredients like berries, dark leafy greens, and nuts play a crucial role in overall health by reducing oxidative stress and inflammation. This is particularly important for diabetics, as oxidative stress is linked to many of the complications associated with diabetes, such as cardiovascular disease and nerve damage. Thus, smoothies not only provide nutritional benefits but also contribute to long-term health maintenance, making them a highly beneficial addition to a diabetic's dietary regimen.

How to Use This Cookbook

Embarking on a journey through the "Diabetic Smoothie Cookbook 2024" offers a refreshing approach to managing diabetes with a delightful twist. The essence of this cookbook lies in its blend of culinary creativity and nutritional science, specifically tailored for those looking to stabilize their blood sugar levels through delicious, wholesome smoothies. Each recipe has been meticulously formulated to ensure that it meets the dietary requirements necessary for a diabetic-friendly diet, focusing on low glycemic index fruits, fibers, and healthy fats.

As you explore the pages of this cookbook, you'll find that it serves not only as a recipe book but also as a guide to understanding how different ingredients can impact your health. This understanding is crucial for making informed choices about the foods you consume. To get the most out of this cookbook, consider how the nutritional content aligns with your specific health needs, taking into account any other medical advice you've received. This awareness will enhance your ability to tailor each smoothie to your personal health goals.

To begin, familiarize yourself with the tools and ingredients recommended in the cookbook. A good blender is essential, as it will be your primary tool for creating smoothies. Investing in fresh, high-quality ingredients is equally important; these form the basis of the nutritious blends you'll be making. Fresh fruits, vegetables, and sources of protein like Greek yogurt or silken tofu can be used to enrich the smoothies, making them both nutritious and filling.

Preparing these smoothies is an opportunity to experiment with flavors and textures. Don't hesitate to modify recipes according to your taste preferences and nutritional needs. If a particular smoothie calls for an ingredient you don't enjoy or can't consume, feel free to substitute it with another that provides a similar nutritional value. This flexibility is key to incorporating the smoothie recipes into your daily routine without feeling restricted.

Consistency is another vital aspect of using this cookbook effectively. Regular consumption of these smoothies as part of a balanced diet can help manage blood sugar levels more effectively. Consider setting a routine that includes a smoothie for the same meal each day—be it breakfast, lunch, or as a snack—this can help in establishing a consistent eating pattern, which is beneficial for blood sugar control.

Another enriching way to use this cookbook is to track your blood sugar responses to different smoothies. This tracking can offer insights into how your body reacts to certain ingredients, helping you fine-tune your diet further. Over time, this will allow you to create a personalized smoothie repertoire that you not only enjoy but that also stabilizes your blood sugar levels.

Lastly, sharing your experiences with these recipes can be incredibly rewarding. Whether it's exchanging notes with friends, participating in online forums, or even creating a blog, discussing your journey adds a layer of support and community that can be inspiring. It reminds you that you're not alone in your journey to manage diabetes and that many others share similar challenges and triumphs. Through this cookbook, you not only nourish your body but also connect with a community, making the path to wellness both enjoyable and supported.

Chapter: 1 Smoothie Basics

Equipment Needed

For anyone diving into the "Diabetic Smoothie Cookbook 2024," having the right equipment is as crucial as the ingredients themselves. The cornerstone of smoothie preparation is a high-quality blender. This tool needs to be powerful enough to handle a variety of ingredients including fibrous vegetables, frozen fruits, and nuts. Blenders with high wattage motors and sharp, durable blades can effortlessly create a smooth texture, ensuring that all the fiber and nutrients are retained without any chunky residue, which is essential for both taste and health.

A variety of blenders are available, ranging from high-performance models to more budget-friendly options. For those who make smoothies regularly, investing in a high-performance blender like those from Vitamix or Blendtec may be worthwhile, as these can handle daily use and maintain a smoother consistency. However, more economical brands also offer models that are sufficient for the average user, though they might require more liquid to process hard ingredients smoothly.

In addition to a blender, having a set of reliable measuring cups and spoons is important. Precise measurement of ingredients is key to ensuring that the nutritional content matches what is specified in the recipes. This precision is particularly important for managing blood sugar levels, as it helps in maintaining consistency in carbohydrate intake. A kitchen scale can also be an invaluable tool for those who prefer to measure ingredients by weight, which can be more accurate than volume measurements.

A spatula may seem like a simple tool, but it is indispensable for ensuring all ingredients are blended thoroughly. It helps in scraping down the sides of the blender jar to make sure everything is incorporated into the smoothie. This is especially useful when blending thicker ingredients like yogurt or peanut butter, which tend to stick to the sides of the blender jar.

For those who like to enjoy their smoothie on the go, investing in some high-quality, insulated smoothie cups or mason jars with tight-sealing lids can be a game changer. These containers not only keep smoothies cold and fresh but also make it easy to carry them to work, the gym, or while running errands. Ensuring the containers are BPA-free is also crucial for health, as it prevents chemicals from leaching into the smoothie.

Another useful addition to your smoothie-making toolkit could be a fine mesh strainer or cheesecloth. These tools come in handy for anyone who prefers their smoothies completely free of pulp or seeds. While most high-quality blenders should eliminate most solid particles, a strainer can ensure a perfectly smooth texture, which can be particularly appealing for those with texture sensitivities.

Finally, for those who enjoy experimenting with flavors and textures, a variety of molds or ice cube trays can be useful for freezing fresh juice, yogurt, or milk into cubes. This allows for a quick and easy way to chill and thicken smoothies without diluting them as regular ice would. Freezing some ingredients ahead of time not only saves preparation time but also enhances the smoothie's texture, making it more enjoyable to drink. With this suite of equipment, anyone can maximize the benefits and enjoyment of the recipes found in the "Diabetic Smoothie Cookbook 2024."

Choosing the Right Ingredients

Selecting the right ingredients is fundamental when preparing diabetic-friendly smoothies, as each choice impacts blood sugar levels, nutritional content, and overall health. Fruits, often a primary ingredient in smoothies, require careful selection; it's advisable to opt for those with a lower glycemic index to avoid rapid spikes in blood sugar. Berries such as blueberries, strawberries, and blackberries, along with apples and pears with their skins on, provide fiber, vitamins, and antioxidants while keeping sugar levels more stable.

Vegetables are another cornerstone for creating nutrient-rich smoothies that support diabetic health. Incorporating greens like spinach, kale, and Swiss chard is beneficial as they are high in fiber and low in carbohydrates. They also add essential vitamins and minerals without significantly altering the flavor of your smoothie. For those looking to add creaminess and additional nutrients, avocados are an excellent choice, packed with healthy fats and a very low carbohydrate content that can help manage blood sugar levels.

Proteins are crucial in managing satiety and stabilizing blood glucose levels. Including a source of protein in your smoothies can transform them from a quick drink to a meal replacement. Good options include Greek yogurt, silken tofu, and nut butters like almond or peanut butter. These ingredients add depth and texture to smoothies while providing the essential amino acids necessary for overall health.

Fats are equally important and should be included in moderation to help absorb vitamins and provide energy. Sources of healthy fats like flaxseeds, chia seeds, and hemp seeds not only increase the nutritional profile of smoothies but also contribute to the feeling of fullness after consumption. These fats are not only beneficial for heart health but can also aid in the slow digestion and absorption of carbohydrates.

Sweeteners should be used sparingly. Natural sweeteners like stevia or monk fruit extract can provide the sweetness that many desire without adding significant calories or affecting blood sugar levels dramatically. It's important to avoid high-glycemic and calorie-dense sweeteners like honey or maple syrup, which can lead to undesirable glucose spikes.

Beyond taste and nutritional content, the texture of smoothies is important and can be enhanced with various thickeners that don't spike blood sugar. Ingredients like oat bran, chia seeds, or even a small portion of rolled oats can improve the smoothie's consistency while adding fiber, which helps slow down the absorption of sugars and maintains a steady blood sugar level.

Lastly, the inclusion of spices and flavor enhancers like cinnamon, vanilla extract, or cocoa powder can make smoothies more enjoyable without adding extra sugars or fats. Cinnamon, in particular, is noted for its potential to lower blood sugar levels and enhance the flavor profile of diabetic-friendly recipes. Each ingredient chosen for a smoothie should not only satisfy taste preferences but also contribute to the nutritional goals of managing diabetes, making each smoothie a tailor-made solution for health and enjoyment.

Tips for Healthy Smoothie Preparation

When embarking on the journey of crafting smoothies from the "Diabetic Smoothie Cookbook 2024," it's essential to start with the selection of the right ingredients. Focusing on fresh, whole foods that are low on the glycemic index is paramount. This includes berries, cherries, apples, and pears, which provide natural sweetness without causing a significant spike in blood sugar levels. Incorporating greens such as spinach or kale not only adds a burst of nutrients but also helps in balancing the natural sugars from the fruits.

The choice of liquid for your smoothies is equally crucial. Opt for water, unsweetened almond milk, or coconut water instead of fruit juices, which can be high in sugars and may affect blood glucose control. These alternatives provide the necessary fluid to achieve the desired smoothie consistency while keeping the carbohydrate content in check. Additionally, the use of dairy or soy milk can offer a creamy texture along with a dose of protein, which is beneficial for blood sugar stabilization.

Adding protein to your smoothies is a smart way to enhance their nutritional value and impact on blood sugar levels. Ingredients like Greek yogurt, silken tofu, or a scoop of protein powder not only make your smoothie more filling but also help slow the absorption of sugars into the bloodstream. This helps in maintaining steadier glucose levels over time, making these smoothies a reliable option for meal replacement or a substantial snack.

Don't overlook the importance of healthy fats in your smoothies, which can further assist in blood sugar management. Avocados, chia seeds, flaxseeds, or a tablespoon of nut butter can add heart-healthy fats that increase satiety and provide a smooth, rich texture to your drink. These fats are not only essential for overall health but also slow the digestion process, which can prevent blood sugar spikes.

The preparation process itself should be mindful. Start by adding the liquids to your blender first, followed by softer ingredients like fresh fruits or yogurt, and finally add harder items such as frozen fruits, ice, or nuts. This sequence ensures that the blender works more efficiently, creating a smoother consistency and preventing wear and tear on the blender's motor.

Experimentation with spices and natural flavor enhancers can transform your smoothies without adding extra sugar or calories. Spices like cinnamon, nutmeg, or ginger can add a punch of flavor and have the added benefit of boosting metabolism or improving insulin sensitivity. Likewise, a dash of vanilla extract or unsweetened cocoa powder can enrich the flavor profile of your smoothie without undermining your glycemic control.

Finally, consider the timing of your smoothie consumption as part of your overall dietary plan. Consuming a smoothie at a time when your body needs more energy, such as before or after a workout, or as a meal replacement when you're short on time, can provide a balanced intake of nutrients. However, it's important to keep portion sizes in check as it's easy to overconsume when drinking your calories. By measuring ingredients and being mindful of the total volume, you can enjoy these nutritious smoothies while effectively managing your diabetes.

Chapter: 2 Breakfast Smoothies

Berry Oat Breakfast Smoothie

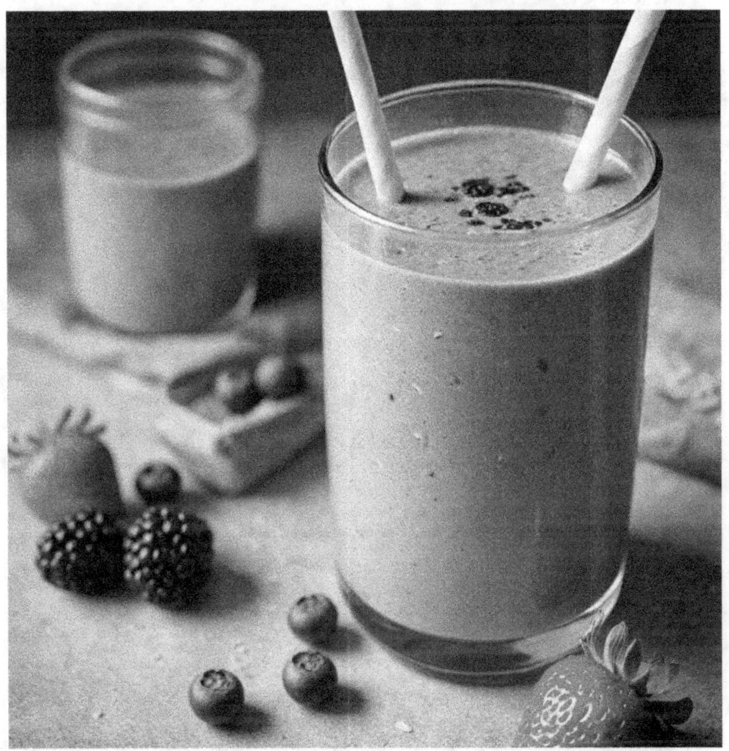

To prepare the Berry Oat Breakfast Smoothie, you will need the following ingredients:

- 1/2 cup of rolled oats
- 1 cup of mixed berries (such as blueberries, strawberries, and raspberries), fresh or frozen
- 1/2 banana, sliced
- 1 tablespoon of chia seeds
- 1 cup of unsweetened almond milk
- A pinch of cinnamon (optional, for extra flavor)

Instructions for making the smoothie are straightforward:

1. Begin by soaking the rolled oats and chia seeds in almond milk for at least 5 minutes. This softens them up and makes the smoothie texture smoother.
2. Place the soaked oats and chia seeds, along with the almond milk, into a blender.
3. Add the mixed berries, banana, and a pinch of cinnamon to the blender.
4. Blend all the ingredients on high until the mixture is smooth and creamy. If the smoothie is too thick, you can add a bit more almond milk to adjust the consistency.
5. Pour the smoothie into a glass and enjoy immediately.

The nutritional information for this smoothie is particularly favorable for

those monitoring their sugar intake. Each serving contains approximately:

- Calories: 300
- Protein: 8 grams
- Fat: 5 grams
- Carbohydrates: 53 grams
- Fiber: 9 grams
- Sugars: 20 grams (from natural sources)

Serving size is crucial, especially for diabetic meal planning. This recipe serves one, making it easy to manage portions and know exactly what you're consuming. The preparation and **cooking time** is minimal, approximately 10 minutes in total, making it a quick and easy option for a busy morning.

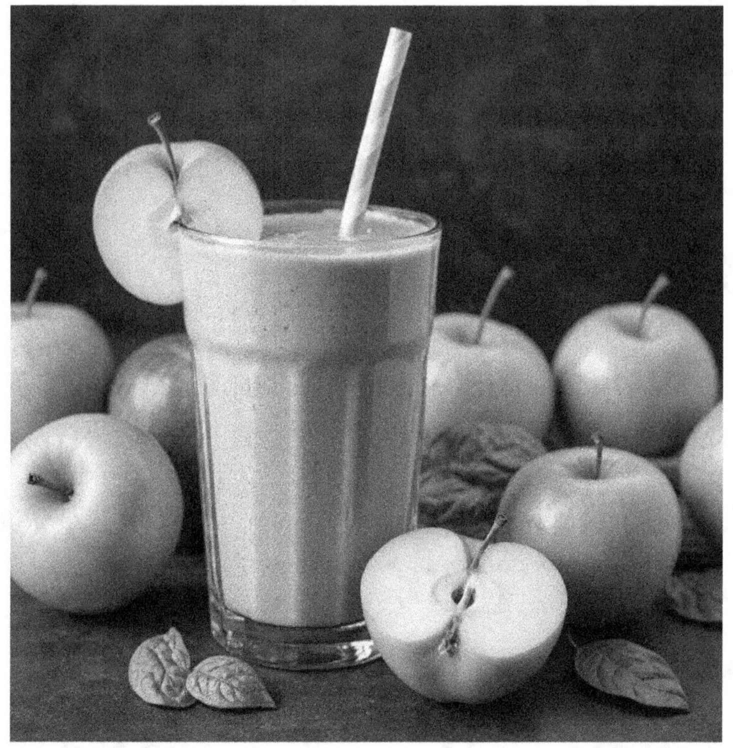

Ingredients for Green Apple Spinach Smoothie:

- 1 large green apple, cored and chopped
- 2 cups fresh spinach leaves
- 1/2 cup plain Greek yogurt
- 1 tablespoon chia seeds
- 1/2 cup unsweetened almond milk

- 1/2 teaspoon ground cinnamon
- Ice cubes (optional, for added chill and thickness)

Instructions:

1. Place the chopped green apple and spinach leaves in the blender.
2. Add the Greek yogurt and chia seeds.
3. Pour in the unsweetened almond milk; this will help the ingredients blend smoothly.
4. Add the ground cinnamon for a hint of spice.
5. If a colder or thicker consistency is desired, add ice cubes.
6. Blend on high speed until all the components are thoroughly combined and the mixture is smooth. Adjust the consistency by adding more almond milk or ice, if necessary.

Nutritional Information:

- Calories: 180
- Carbohydrates: 28g
- Fiber: 6g
- Protein: 8g
- Fat: 4g
- Sugar: 15g (natural sugars from the apple and a small amount from yogurt)

Serving Size:

- This recipe yields approximately one 16-ounce serving, ideal for one person as a complete breakfast meal.

Cooking Time:

- The total preparation and blending time is about 5 minutes, making this smoothie a quick and easy option for busy mornings.

Cinnamon Roll Smoothie

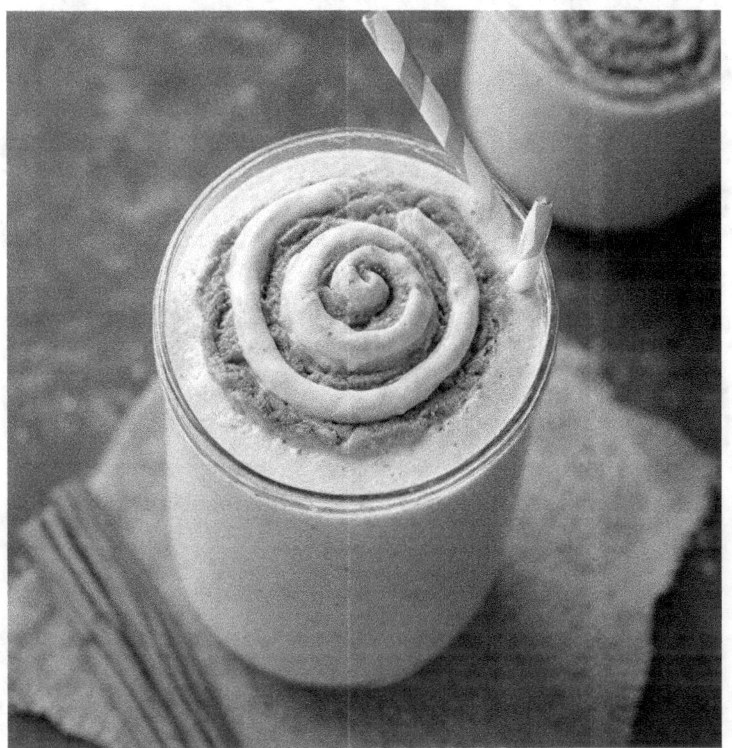

Ingredients:

- 1/2 cup unsweetened almond milk
- 1/4 cup Greek yogurt, plain
- 1 small banana, frozen
- 2 tablespoons rolled oats
- 1 tablespoon chia seeds
- 1 teaspoon ground cinnamon

- 1/4 teaspoon vanilla extract
- Ice cubes (optional, for a thicker smoothie)
- Optional sweetener: 1 teaspoon of stevia or monk fruit sweetener

Instructions:

1. Place the almond milk and Greek yogurt in the blender as the base to ensure smooth blending.
2. Add the frozen banana and rolled oats next; these provide the smoothie's body and creamy texture.
3. Follow with chia seeds for fiber, which aids in blood sugar regulation.
4. Sprinkle in the ground cinnamon and add vanilla extract for that classic cinnamon roll flavor.
5. Blend on high until smooth. If the consistency is too thick, adjust by adding a little more almond milk.
6. Taste and add stevia or monk fruit sweetener if a sweeter smoothie is desired.
7. Serve immediately for the best texture and flavor.

Nutritional Information:

- Calories: 250
- Carbohydrates: 38g
- Fiber: 7g
- Sugars: 15g (natural sugars from the banana)
- Protein: 10g

- Fat: 6g

Serving Size:

- This recipe yields one serving, ideal for a filling and nutritious single breakfast meal.

Cooking Time:

- Preparation time is about 5 minutes. No cooking is required, just blending, making it perfect for a quick and easy diabetic-friendly breakfast.

Avocado Berry Smoothie

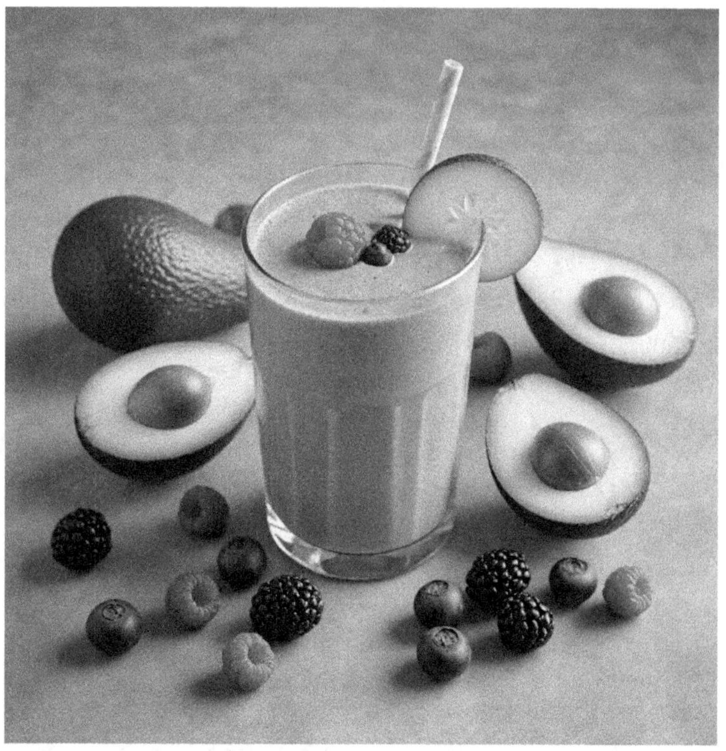

Ingredients:

- 1/2 ripe avocado
- 1/2 cup mixed berries (such as blueberries, raspberries, and strawberries), fresh or frozen
- 1 cup spinach leaves
- 1 tablespoon chia seeds
- 1 cup unsweetened almond milk

- A pinch of cinnamon (optional)

Instructions:

1. Place the almond milk in the blender first, which will help in achieving a smoother blend.

2. Add the spinach leaves and chia seeds next, ensuring they are submerged for better processing.

3. Scoop in the avocado and add the mixed berries.

4. Sprinkle a pinch of cinnamon for an extra flavor boost, if desired.

5. Blend on high for about 30 seconds or until the mixture is smooth and creamy. If the smoothie is too thick, you can add a little more almond milk to adjust the consistency to your liking.

Nutritional Information:

- Calories: 290
- Carbohydrates: 24g
- Fiber: 10g
- Sugars: 8g
- Protein: 5g
- Fat: 19g

Serving Size:

- This recipe yields one serving, making it a quick and easy option for a busy morning.

Cooking Time:

- Total preparation and blending time is approximately 5 minutes, making it an efficient choice for those who need a nutritious breakfast that fits into a hectic schedule.

Incorporating this Avocado Berry Smoothie into your morning routine is a fantastic way to support your dietary needs without compromising on taste or texture. The blend of avocado and berries not only provides essential nutrients but also helps in maintaining glycemic control, crucial for those managing diabetes. This recipe exemplifies how the cookbook provides practical, tasty solutions for a diabetic-friendly diet, emphasizing the importance of enjoying what you eat while taking good care of your health.

Peanut Butter Banana Smoothie

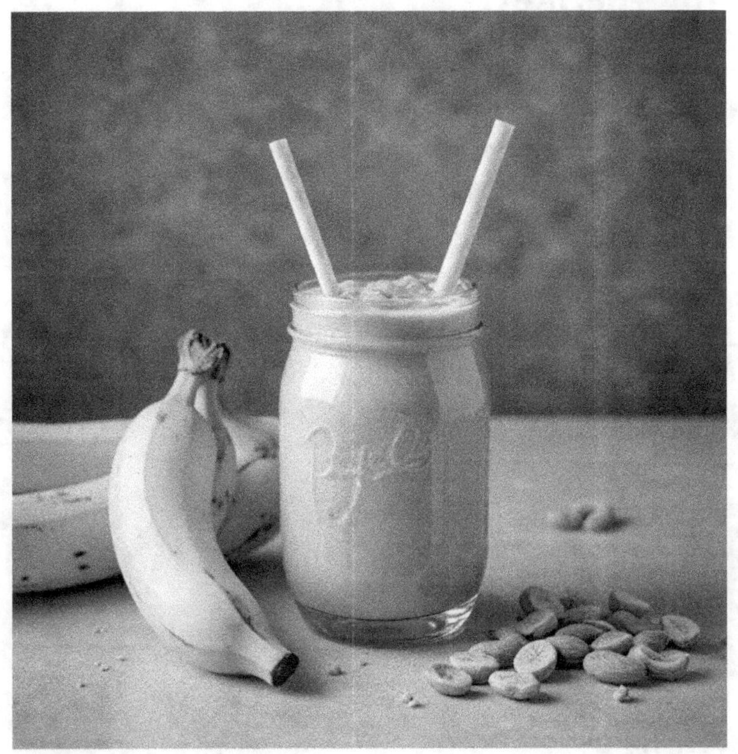

Ingredients:

- 1 medium ripe banana, frozen
- 2 tablespoons unsweetened peanut butter
- 1 cup unsweetened almond milk
- 1/2 teaspoon vanilla extract
- 1 tablespoon flaxseeds
- Ice cubes (optional, for thicker consistency)

Instructions:

1. Place the frozen banana, peanut butter, almond milk, and vanilla extract into the blender.
2. Add the flaxseeds, which provide an additional layer of nutrients and help thicken the smoothie.
3. Blend on high speed until the mixture is smooth and creamy. If the smoothie is too thick, add more almond milk to achieve the desired consistency.
4. If preferred, add a few ice cubes to the blender and pulse until well mixed and frosty.

Nutritional Information:

- Calories: 330
- Carbohydrates: 38g
- Fiber: 6g
- Protein: 10g
- Fat: 18g
- Sugars: 17g

Serving Size: This recipe yields about 1 serving (approximately 16 oz).

Cooking Time: The total preparation time, including blending, is about 5 minutes.

Carrot Cake Smoothie

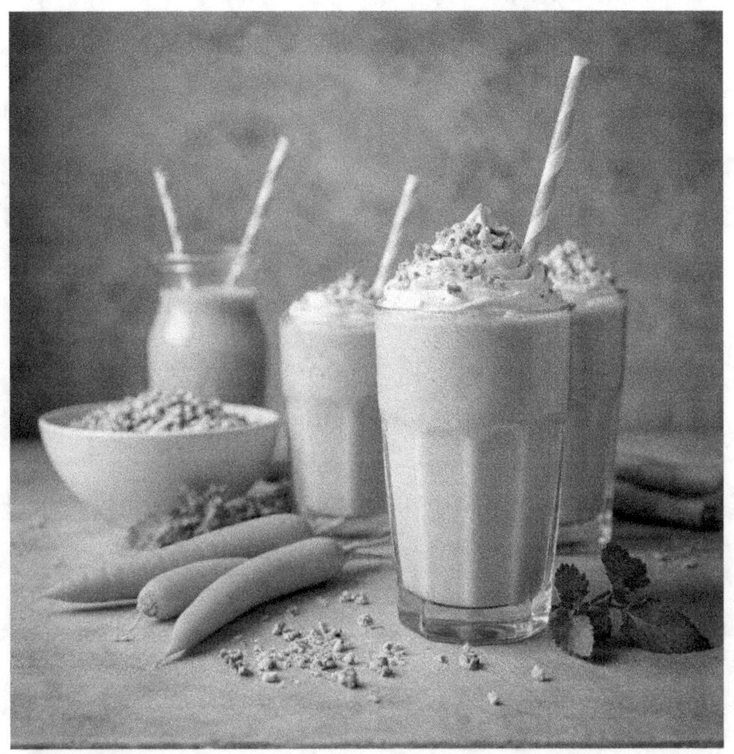

Ingredients:

- 1/2 cup chopped carrots
- 1/4 cup rolled oats
- 2 tablespoons chopped walnuts
- 1 tablespoon chia seeds
- 1/2 teaspoon cinnamon
- 1/4 teaspoon nutmeg

- 1 cup unsweetened almond milk

- 1/2 frozen banana

- Optional: a pinch of stevia or a small amount of maple syrup for extra sweetness

Instructions:

1. Begin by soaking the rolled oats and chia seeds in the almond milk for at least ten minutes; this process will soften them and make the smoothie creamier.

2. Place the softened oats and chia seeds, along with the rest of the ingredients, into a blender.

3. Blend on high until the mixture reaches a smooth and creamy consistency. If the smoothie is too thick, add a bit more almond milk to adjust the texture.

4. Taste and add a pinch of stevia or a drizzle of maple syrup if a sweeter smoothie is desired.

Nutritional Information:

- Calories: Approximately 300

- Carbohydrates: 35g

- Fiber: 8g

- Sugars: 12g (natural sugars from the banana and carrots)

- Protein: 8g

- Fat: 15g (healthy fats from walnuts and chia seeds)

Serving Size:

This recipe makes one serving, perfect for a filling and nutritious single breakfast meal.

Cooking Time:

The preparation and blending time is around 15 minutes, making it a quick and convenient option for a busy morning.

Coconut Almond Smoothie

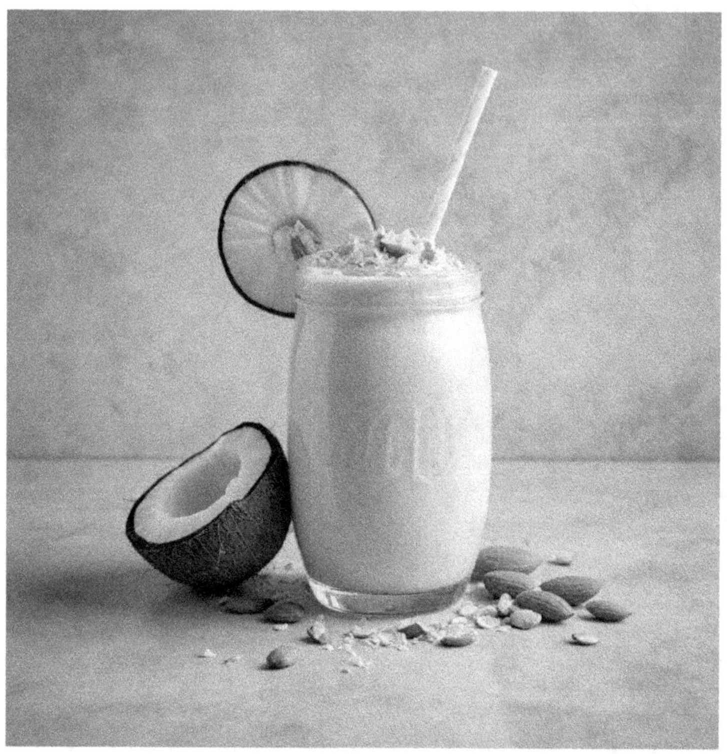

Ingredients:

- 1 cup unsweetened almond milk
- 1/2 cup Greek yogurt, plain
- 1/4 cup shredded unsweetened coconut
- 2 tablespoons almond butter
- 1 tablespoon chia seeds
- 1/2 teaspoon vanilla extract

- Ice cubes (optional, for thicker consistency.

Instructions:

1. Start by adding the almond milk to the blender to facilitate smoother blending.
2. Add the Greek yogurt and almond butter, ensuring they blend evenly with the milk, creating a creamy base.
3. Incorporate the shredded coconut, chia seeds, and vanilla extract, blending again until the mixture achieves a uniform, smooth texture. If a thicker consistency is desired, add a few ice cubes and blend until smooth.
4. Pour the smoothie into a glass and, if desired, sprinkle a little extra coconut on top for garnish.

Nutritional Information:

- Calories: 380
- Total Fat: 28g
- Saturated Fat: 10g
- Carbohydrates: 18g
- Fiber: 6g
- Sugars: 7g
- Protein: 15g

Serving Size: This recipe yields one serving.

Cooking Time: Preparation takes approximately 5 minutes.

Mango Chia Seed Smoothie

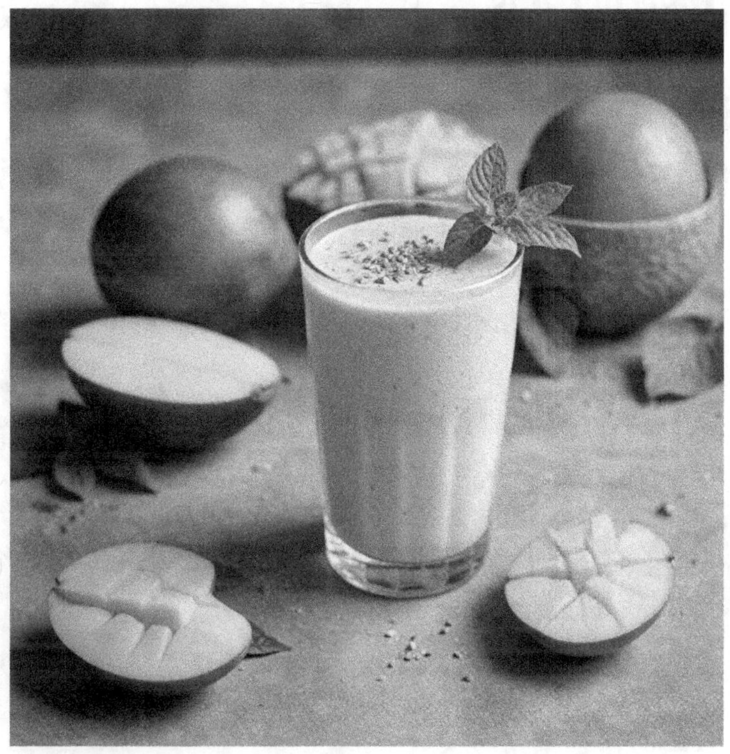

Ingredients:

- 1 cup fresh mango chunks
- 1 tablespoon chia seeds
- 1/2 cup unsweetened almond milk
- 1/2 cup Greek yogurt, plain
- 1/4 teaspoon vanilla extract
- Ice cubes (optional, for a thicker smoothie)

Instructions:

1. In a blender, combine the mango chunks and unsweetened almond milk. Blend until the mango is pureed.
2. Add the Greek yogurt, chia seeds, and vanilla extract. If a thicker consistency is preferred, add a few ice cubes.
3. Blend everything together until smooth. If the smoothie is too thick, adjust by adding a little more almond milk until the desired consistency is achieved.

Nutritional Information:

Each serving of the Mango Chia Seed Smoothie provides approximately:
- Calories: 200
- Carbohydrates: 28 g
- Fiber: 5 g
- Protein: 8 g
- Fat: 6 g
- Sodium: 50 mg

Serving Size:

This recipe yields about 2 cups, serving 1 or 2 people depending on portion preference.

Cooking Time:

The total time required to prepare and blend this smoothie is about 5 minutes.

Peach and Cottage Cheese Smoothie

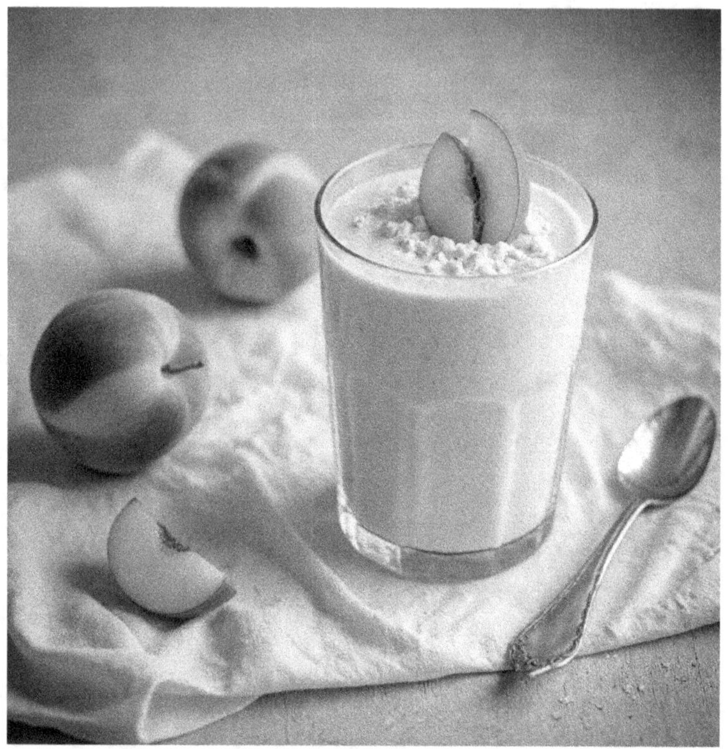

Ingredient List:

- 1 cup fresh or frozen peach slices
- 1/2 cup low-fat cottage cheese
- 1/4 teaspoon ground cinnamon
- 1 tablespoon chia seeds
- 1/2 cup unsweetened almond milk
- Ice cubes (optional, for a thicker consistency)

Instructions:

1. Place all ingredients in a blender, starting with the almond milk to facilitate smoother blending.

2. Blend on high until smooth and creamy. Add a few ice cubes if a thicker consistency is desired and blend again until smooth.

3. Pour into a glass and enjoy immediately for the best flavor and nutrient retention.

Nutritional Information:

- Calories: 210
- Total Fat: 4g
- Saturated Fat: 1g
- Carbohydrates: 30g
- Fiber: 5g
- Sugars: 20g (natural sugars from peach)
- Protein: 14g

Serving Size:

- This recipe yields one serving, perfect for a filling single breakfast meal.

Cooking Time:

- Prep time: 5 minutes
- Blend time: 2 minutes

- Total time: 7 minutes

Vanilla Latte Smoothie

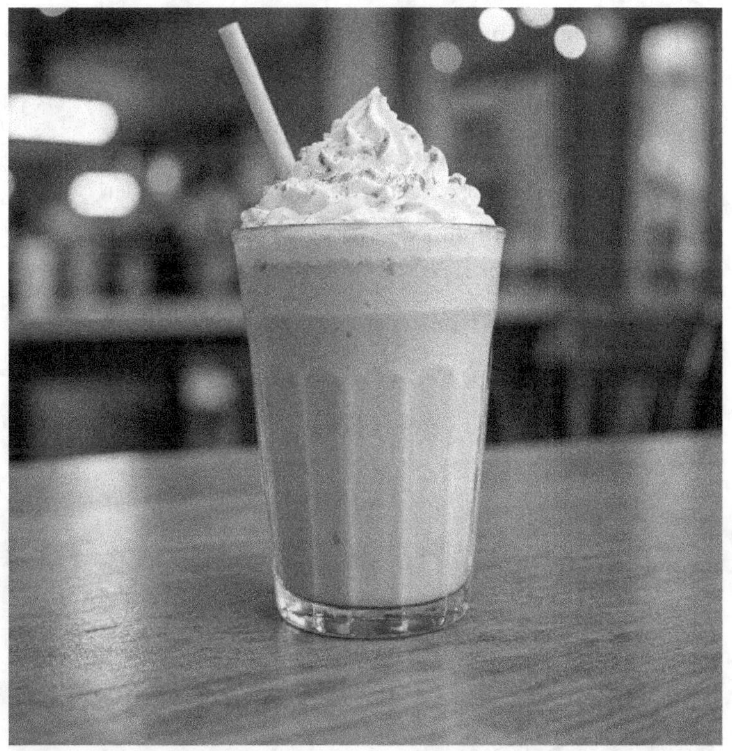

Ingredients:

- 1/2 cup unsweetened almond milk

- 1/2 cup brewed coffee, cooled

- 1/4 cup Greek yogurt, plain

- 1 teaspoon vanilla extract

- 1 tablespoon chia seeds

- 1 tablespoon almond butter

- 1/2 teaspoon ground cinnamon
- Ice cubes (optional, for thicker consistency)
- Stevia or monk fruit sweetener to taste

Instructions:

1. Place all ingredients except the ice cubes into a blender.
2. Blend on high until smooth. If a thicker consistency is desired, add ice cubes and blend again.
3. Taste and adjust sweetness with stevia or monk fruit sweetener as needed.

Nutritional Information:

- Calories: 190
- Total Fat: 11g (Saturated Fat: 1g)
- Carbohydrates: 13g (Fiber: 4g, Sugars: 5g)
- Protein: 9g

Serving Size:

- Makes 1 serving

Cooking Time:

- Preparation and blending time: 5 minutes

Chapter: 3 Lunch Smoothies

Tomato Basil Smoothie

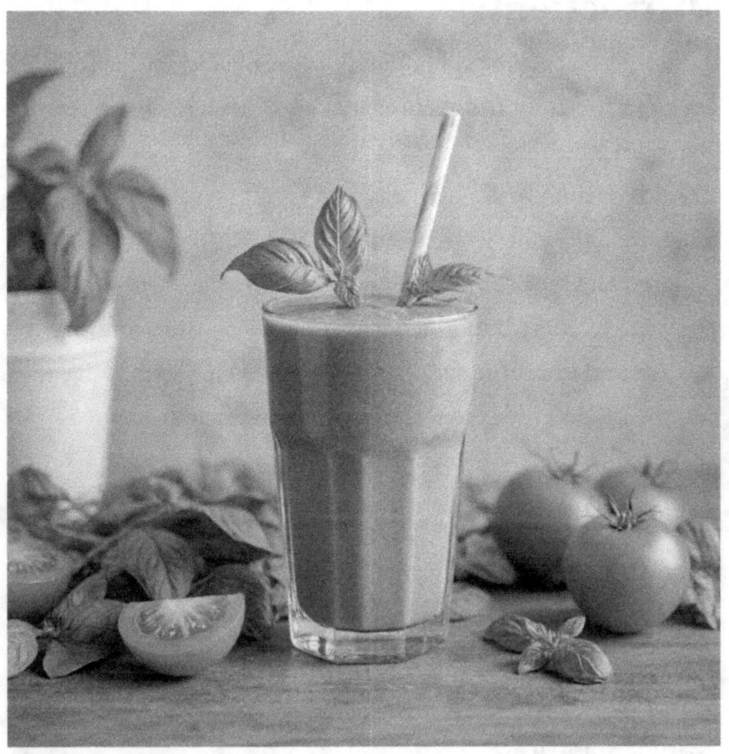

Ingredients:

- 1 cup chopped tomatoes

- 1/2 cup unsweetened almond milk

- 1/4 cup fresh basil leaves

- 1/2 cucumber, peeled and chopped

- 1 tablespoon chia seeds
- 1/4 teaspoon salt
- Ice cubes (optional)

Instructions:

1. Start by placing the almond milk in the blender, followed by the chopped tomatoes and cucumber. This sequence helps in creating a smoother blend.
2. Add the fresh basil, chia seeds, and salt. If you prefer a chilled smoothie, add a few ice cubes at this stage.
3. Blend on high until all the ingredients are thoroughly combined and the smoothie achieves a smooth, even consistency.
4. Taste and adjust the seasoning if necessary. If the smoothie is too thick, add a little more almond milk to reach the desired consistency

Nutritional Information:

- Calories: 120
- Total Fat: 4g
- Saturated Fat: 0.5g
- Cholesterol: 0mg
- Sodium: 300mg
- Total Carbohydrates: 18g
- Dietary Fiber: 5g
- Sugars: 9g (includes 0g added sugars)

- Protein: 4g

Serving Size:

- Makes about 2 cups (serves 1 as a meal or 2 as a snack).

Cooking Time:

- Prep time: 5 minutes
- Blend time: 2 minutes
- Total time: 7 minutes

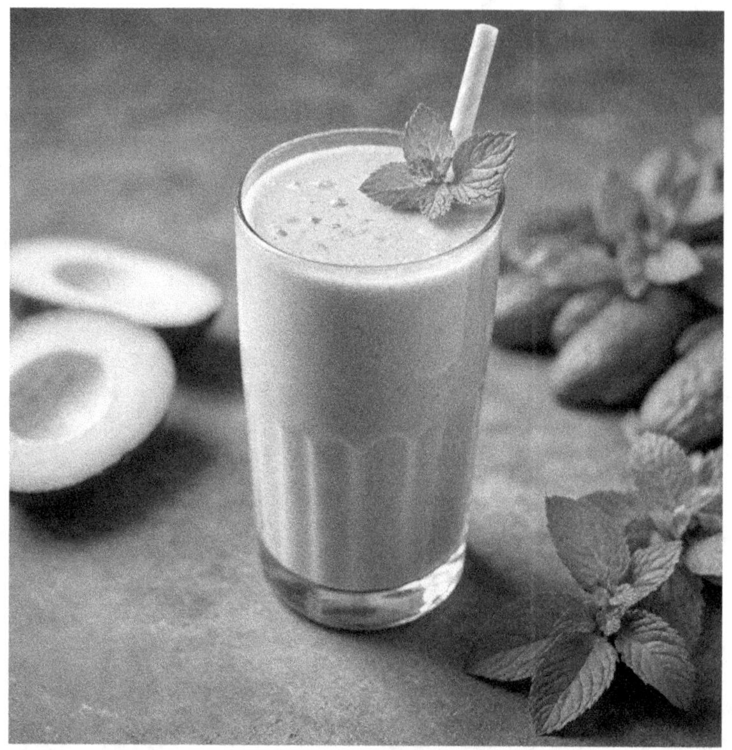

Ingredients for Cucumber Mint Refresh Smoothie:

- 1 large cucumber, peeled and chopped
- 1/2 cup of fresh mint leaves
- 1/2 cup of Greek yogurt (unsweetened)
- 1 tablespoon of lemon juice
- 1/2 cup of ice cubes

- 1 tablespoon of chia seeds
- Optional: Stevia or another non-nutritive sweetener, to taste

Instructions:

1. Place the cucumber, mint leaves, and lemon juice into the blender.
2. Add the Greek yogurt and ice cubes on top to help weigh down the lighter ingredients for better blending.
3. Blend on high until the mixture becomes smooth.
4. Add the chia seeds and blend again briefly just to mix them through evenly.
5. Taste the smoothie and, if needed, add a small amount of non-nutritive sweetener to enhance the sweetness.

Nutritional Information:

Each serving of the Cucumber Mint Refresh Smoothie provides approximately:
- Calories: 120
- Carbohydrates: 14g
- Fiber: 3g
- Protein: 6g
- Fat: 3g

This nutritional content is optimal for a diabetic-friendly diet, with a good balance of carbohydrates and protein to help regulate blood sugar levels. The high fiber content also aids in slow digestion and further stabilizes glucose levels.

Serving Size:

This recipe yields about 2 cups, suitable for one large lunch serving or two smaller servings if preferred as a light lunch accompaniment.

Cooking Time:

The total time required to prepare and blend the Cucumber Mint Refresh Smoothie is about 5 minutes, making it a quick and efficient option for a nutritious lunch that doesn't take much time out of your day.

Spiced Pumpkin Smoothie

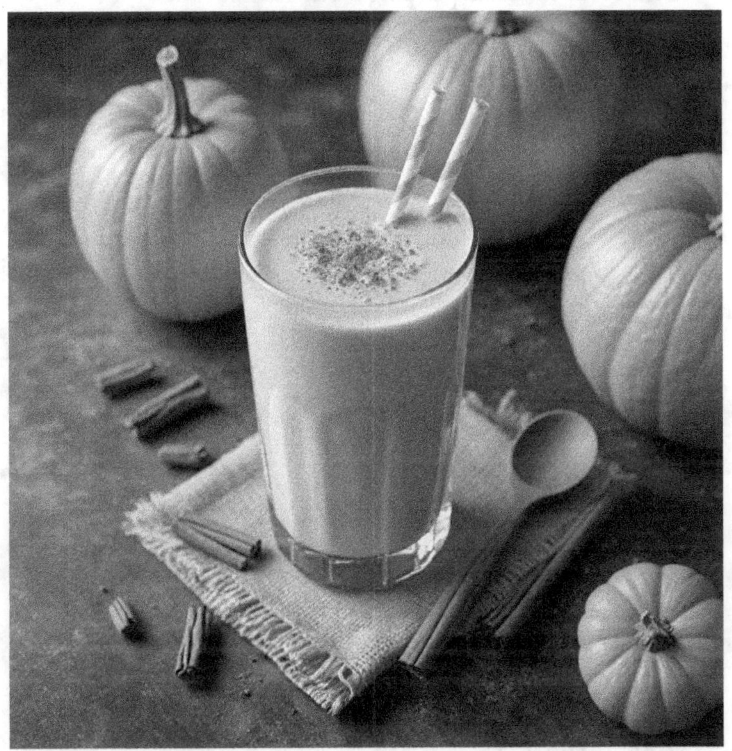

Ingredients:

- 1/2 cup canned pumpkin puree (ensure it's unsweetened)
- 1 cup unsweetened almond milk
- 1/2 banana, slightly ripe (for natural sweetness)
- 1 tablespoon chia seeds (for added fiber and protein)
- 1/2 teaspoon ground cinnamon
- 1/4 teaspoon ground nutmeg

- 1/2 teaspoon vanilla extract
- Ice cubes (optional, depending on desired thickness)

Instructions:

1. Place the pumpkin puree, almond milk, and banana into the blender.
2. Add the chia seeds, cinnamon, nutmeg, and vanilla extract.
3. Blend on high until all the ingredients are well combined and the mixture is smooth.
4. If the smoothie is too thick, adjust the consistency by adding a little more almond milk. If it's too thin, add a few ice cubes and blend again to thicken.
5. Pour into a glass and enjoy immediately for the best taste and nutrient retention.

Nutritional Information:

- Calories: 185
- Carbohydrates: 27g
- Fiber: 7g
- Protein: 4g
- Fat: 5g
- Sugar: 12g

Serving Size: This recipe yields approximately 1 serving.

Cooking Time: The total preparation time is about 5 minutes, making it a quick and easy option for a busy midday meal.

Zesty Orange Carrot Smoothie

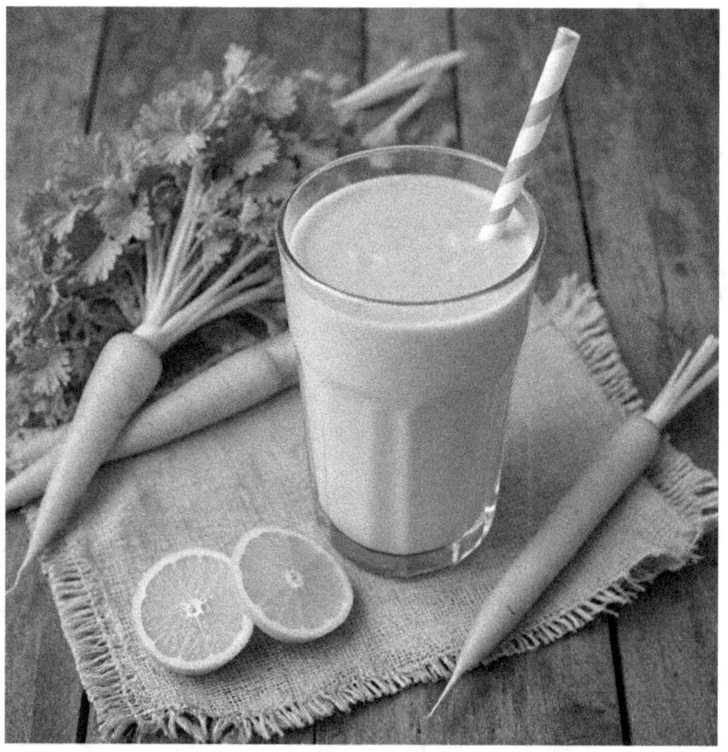

Ingredients:

- 1 large carrot, peeled and chopped

- 1 orange, peeled and deseeded

- 1/2 inch piece of ginger, peeled

- 1/2 lemon, juiced

- 1 tablespoon of flaxseed meal

- 1 cup of water or unsweetened almond milk

- Ice cubes (optional)

Instructions:

1. Start by preparing the ingredients: wash, peel, and chop the carrot; peel and deseed the orange; peel the ginger.
2. Place the carrot, orange, ginger, and lemon juice into the blender. Add the flaxseed meal for an extra boost of fiber and omega-3 fatty acids, which are excellent for heart health.
3. Pour in one cup of water or almond milk to help blend the ingredients smoothly and achieve a creamy texture.
4. Blend on high until all components are thoroughly mixed and the smoothie has a smooth consistency. Add ice cubes if a colder beverage is preferred and blend again.
5. Taste and adjust the flavor as needed, adding more lemon juice or ginger for extra zing.

Nutritional Information (per serving):

- Calories: 150
- Carbohydrates: 29g
- Fiber: 6g
- Protein: 3g
- Fat: 3g
- Sugars: 18g

Serving Size: 1 large glass (about 12 ounces)

Cooking Time: 5 minutes

Bell Pepper and Lemon Smoothie

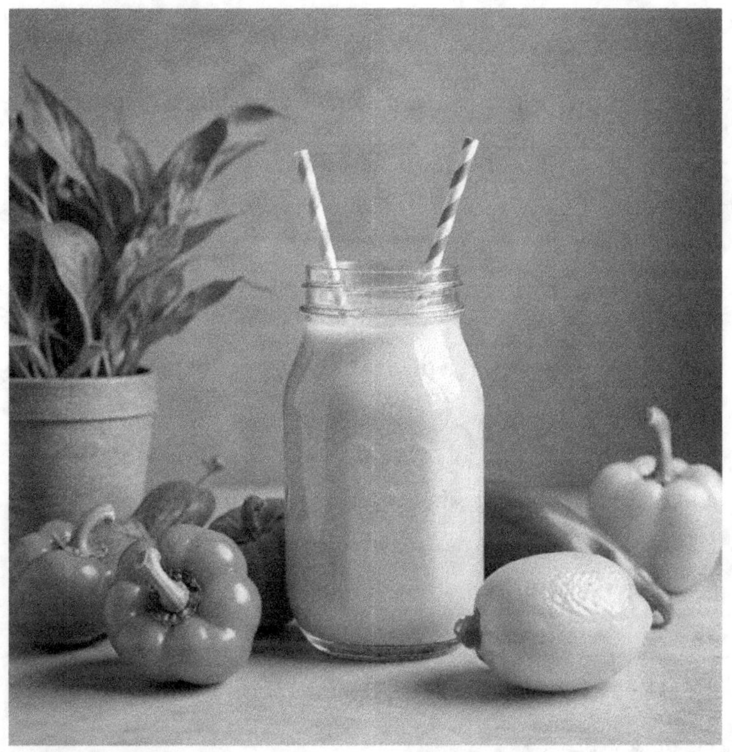

Ingredients:

- 1 red bell pepper, seeded and chopped
- 1 small cucumber, peeled and chopped
- Juice of 1 lemon
- 1 tablespoon of flaxseed, ground
- 1 cup of cold water or unsweetened almond milk
- Ice cubes (optional for thicker consistency)

- A handful of fresh parsley

Instructions:

1. Start by preparing your ingredients: wash and chop the bell pepper and cucumber, and juice the lemon.
2. Place the chopped bell pepper, cucumber, and fresh parsley into the blender.
3. Add the ground flaxseed and the lemon juice to the mix.
4. Pour in one cup of cold water or almond milk to help blend the ingredients smoothly. If a thicker consistency is desired, add a few ice cubes.
5. Blend on high until all the components are thoroughly mixed and the smoothie has a smooth, creamy texture.
6. Taste and adjust the flavor as needed, adding more lemon juice for tartness or water for dilution.

Nutritional Information:

- Calories: 118
- Carbohydrates: 17g
- Fiber: 5g
- Protein: 3g
- Fat: 4g
- Sugar: 10g (Natural sugars from the ingredients)

Serving Size:

- This recipe yields approximately 16 ounces (about 2 cups), serving 1 person as a full meal replacement or 2 people as a light meal accompaniment.

Cooking Time:

- Preparation time: About 10 minutes
- No cooking required

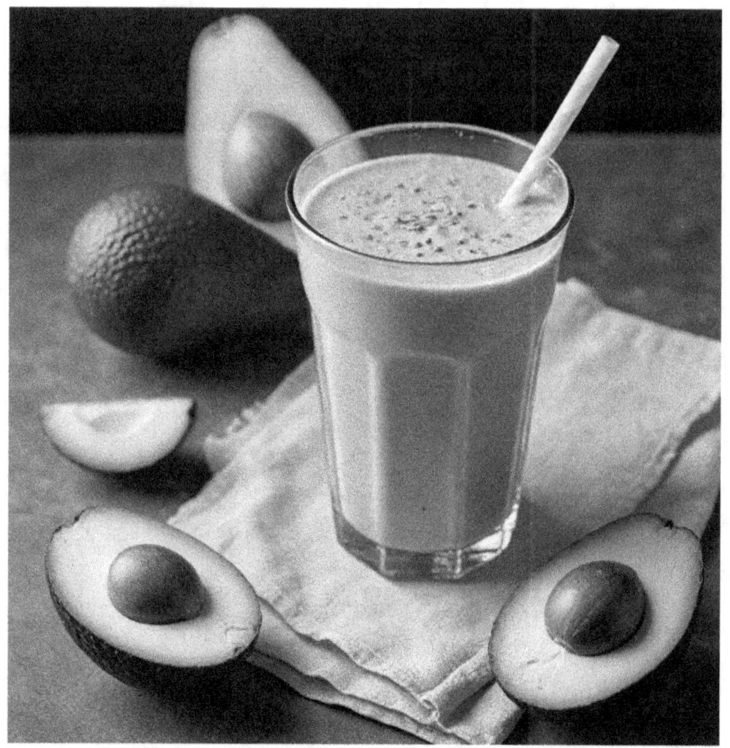

For the Savory Avocado Smoothie, the ingredients required are:

- 1 ripe avocado, peeled and pitted
- 1 cup fresh spinach
- 1 small cucumber, peeled and chopped
- 1/2 cup plain Greek yogurt
- 1/4 cup fresh cilantro

- 1 tablespoon lime juice

- 1 small garlic clove

- Salt and pepper to taste

- 1/2 cup water or unsweetened almond milk for thinning

Instructions to prepare the smoothie are straightforward:

1. Place the avocado, spinach, cucumber, Greek yogurt, cilantro, lime juice, and garlic in the blender.
2. Season with a pinch of salt and pepper.
3. Add water or almond milk to reach the desired consistency.
4. Blend on high until smooth and creamy. Adjust seasoning as needed.
5. Serve immediately to maintain freshness and flavor.

Nutritional information is crucial for those monitoring their intake:

- Calories: Approximately 280
- Carbohydrates: 18g
- Fiber: 7g
- Protein: 8g
- Fat: 20g

This smoothie offers a balance of healthy fats, proteins, and fiber to help regulate blood sugar levels throughout the afternoon.

The **serving size** for the Savory Avocado Smoothie is typically one large glass, which makes it a filling and nutritious option for a meal replacement or a substantial snack.

Cooking time is minimal, making this smoothie an ideal choice for a quick and healthy lunch. From preparation to serving, the total time required is about 5 minutes, allowing even the busiest individuals to enjoy a nutritious meal without significant time commitment.

Tart Cherry Lime Smoothie

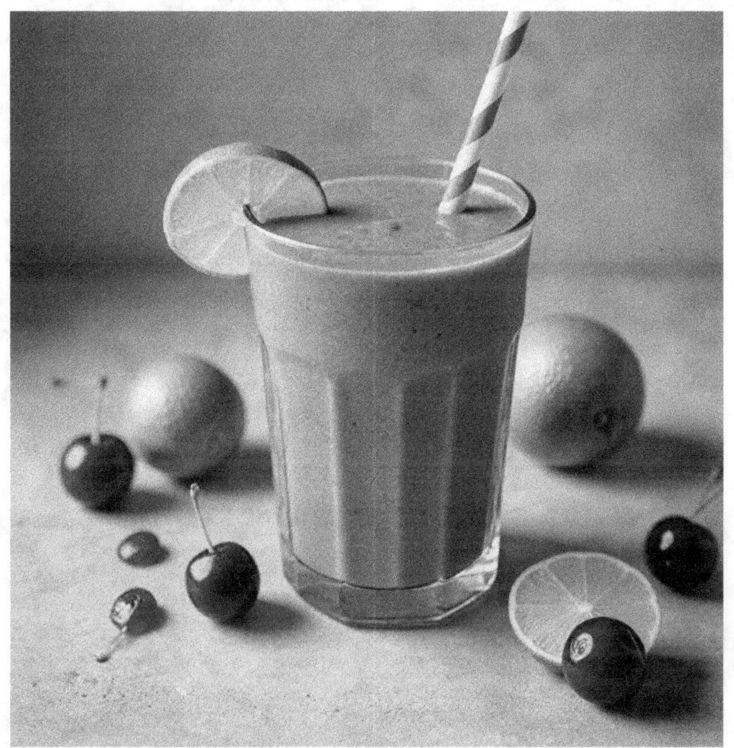

The ingredients needed for this smoothie include:

- 1 cup frozen tart cherries
- Juice of 1 lime
- 1/2 cup unsweetened almond milk
- 1/2 cup Greek yogurt, plain
- 1 tablespoon chia seeds

- A handful of spinach (optional, for added nutrients)
- Ice cubes (optional, for a thicker consistency)

To prepare the Tart Cherry Lime Smoothie, start by placing all ingredients in a blender. Blend on high speed until smooth. If the smoothie is too thick, add a little more almond milk to reach the desired consistency. If more sweetness is desired, consider adding a small amount of stevia or another low-calorie sweetener. Pour into a glass and enjoy immediately to maximize the benefits of the nutrients.

The nutritional information for this smoothie, assuming one serving, is as follows:

- Calories: Approximately 200
- Protein: 10 grams
- Fat: 4 grams
- Carbohydrates: 30 grams
- Dietary Fiber: 5 grams
- Sugars: 20 grams (naturally occurring from cherries and yogurt)

The **serving size** for this recipe is one glass, which is perfect for one person as a meal replacement or a substantial snack. It is important to be mindful of serving sizes, especially when managing dietary intake for diabetes.

The total **preparation time** for the Tart Cherry Lime Smoothie
is about 5 minutes, making it an excellent choice for a quick,
healthful lunch option that doesn't require much time to prepare.
This short cooking time ensures that busy individuals can still
enjoy a nutritious meal even when pressed for time.

Broccoli and Pineapple Medley Smoothie

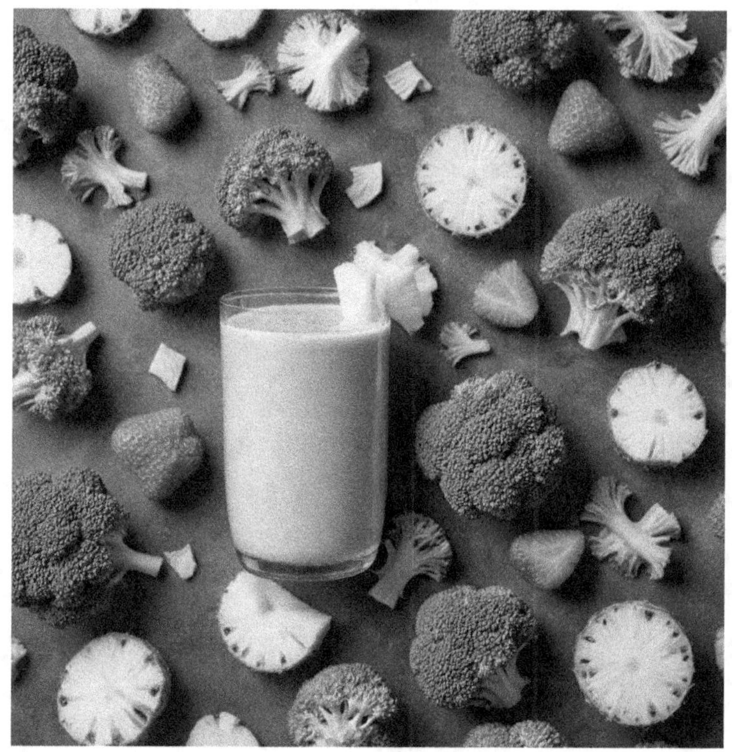

Ingredients for Broccoli and Pineapple Medley Smoothie:

- 1 cup chopped fresh broccoli, stems included
- 1 cup frozen pineapple chunks
- 1/2 banana, sliced

- 1 cup unsweetened almond milk
- 1 tablespoon chia seeds
- 1 scoop vanilla protein powder (optional, for added protein)

Instructions:

1. Start by preparing the broccoli: wash it thoroughly under running water and chop it into small pieces. Include both florets and stems to maximize nutrient intake.

2. Place the chopped broccoli, frozen pineapple chunks, and banana slices into a blender.

3. Add the unsweetened almond milk to help facilitate smoother blending. For a thicker consistency, you can use less almond milk.

4. Add chia seeds for a boost of fiber and omega-3 fatty acids, which are beneficial for heart health.

5. If desired, include a scoop of vanilla protein powder to increase the protein content, which can help with blood sugar stabilization.

6. Blend on high until all the ingredients are thoroughly combined and the smoothie reaches your desired consistency. If the smoothie is too thick, you can add a bit more almond milk and blend again.

7. Pour into a glass and serve immediately.

Nutritional Information:

- Calories: Approximately 280 kcal per serving
- Carbohydrates: 45g

- Fiber: 9g
- Protein: 8g (more if protein powder is added)
- Fat: 7g

Serving Size:

- This recipe yields about 2 cups (16 ounces), serving 1-2 people depending on portion preference.

Cooking Time:

- Total preparation and blending time is about 5 minutes.

Sweet Pea and Mint Smoothie

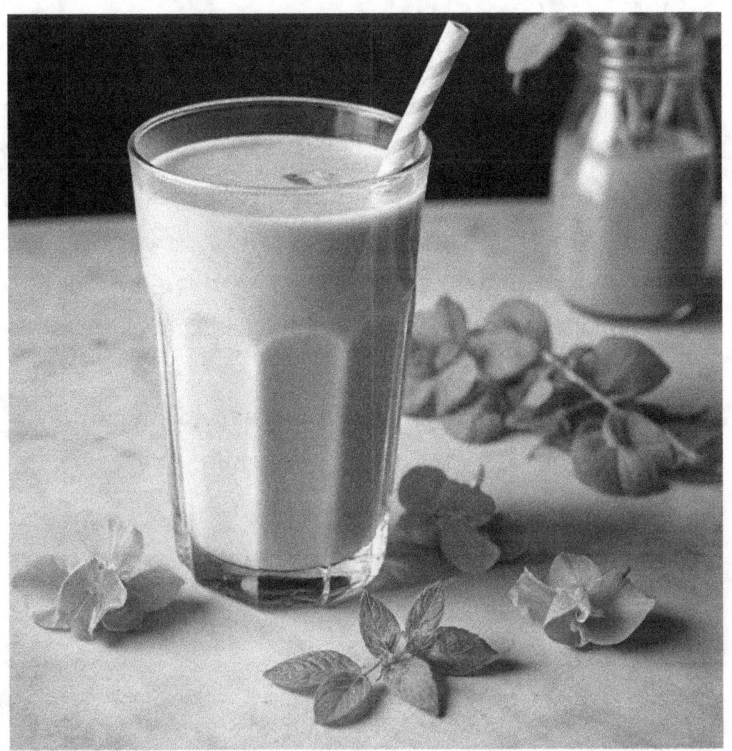

Ingredients:

- 1 cup frozen green peas
- 1/2 cup fresh mint leaves
- 1/2 cucumber, peeled and chopped
- 1/2 cup Greek yogurt, plain and unsweetened
- 1 tablespoon lemon juice
- 1/2 cup water or unsweetened almond milk

- Ice cubes (optional)

Instructions:

1. In a blender, combine the frozen green peas, fresh mint leaves, and chopped cucumber.
2. Add the Greek yogurt and lemon juice to the blender.
3. Pour in the water or almond milk to facilitate blending.
4. Blend on high until the mixture is smooth. If the smoothie is too thick, add a little more water or almond milk to achieve the desired consistency.
5. Add ice cubes if preferred, and blend again until smooth.
6. Serve immediately for the best flavor and nutrient retention.

Nutritional Information (per serving):

- Calories: 150
- Carbohydrates: 22g
- Fiber: 6g
- Protein: 10g
- Fat: 3g
- Sugar: 9g (natural sugars from peas and cucumber)

Serving Size:

- This recipe yields about 2 servings.

Cooking Time:

- Total preparation time is approximately 10 minutes.

Spinach, Kiwi, and Cucumber Smoothie

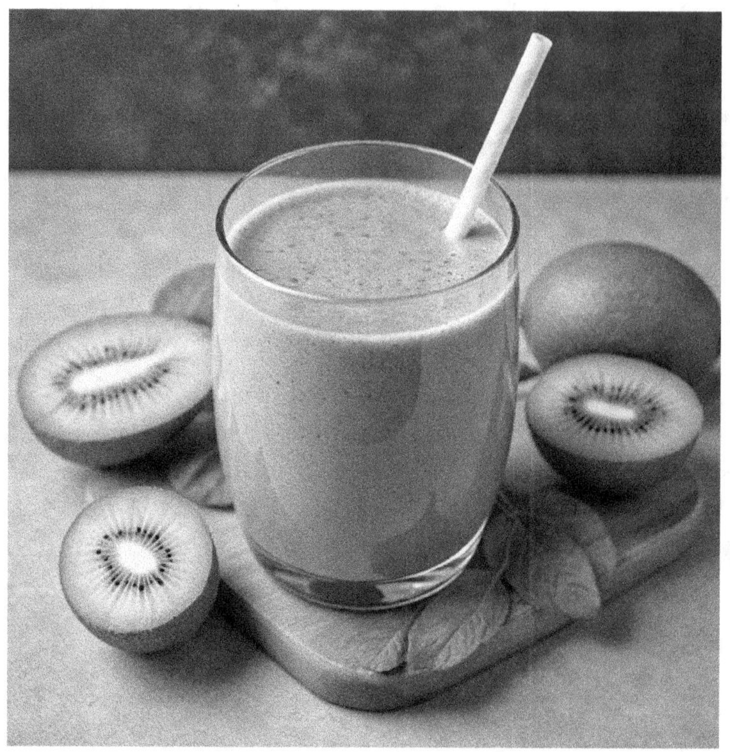

Ingredients:

- Spinach: 1 cup (packed)
- Kiwi: 2 medium, peeled and sliced
- Cucumber: 1 medium, peeled and chopped
- Greek yogurt (unsweetened): 1/2 cup
- Chia seeds: 1 tablespoon
- Water or unsweetened almond milk: 1/2 cup

- Ice cubes: 4-5

Instructions:

1. Begin by preparing your ingredients: wash the spinach leaves, peel and slice the kiwis, and peel and chop the cucumber.
2. In a blender, add the water or almond milk first to facilitate smoother blending.
3. Add the spinach, cucumber, and kiwi slices to the blender.
4. Include the Greek yogurt and chia seeds for a protein and omega-3 boost.
5. Top off with ice cubes.
6. Blend on high until the mixture reaches a smooth, creamy consistency. If the smoothie is too thick, you can add a little more liquid to adjust the consistency to your liking.

Nutritional Information:

- Calories: 210
- Carbohydrates: 30g
- Fiber: 5g
- Protein: 8g
- Fat: 5g
- Sugars: 18g (Natural sugars from fruits)

Serving Size:

This recipe yields approximately 16 ounces (2 cups), suitable for one large serving or two smaller servings, making it ideal for a fulfilling lunch portion.

Cooking Time:

Total preparation and blending time is about 10 minutes, making it a quick and easy option for a busy day.

Chapter:4 Dinner Smoothies

Roasted Beet and Ginger Smoothie

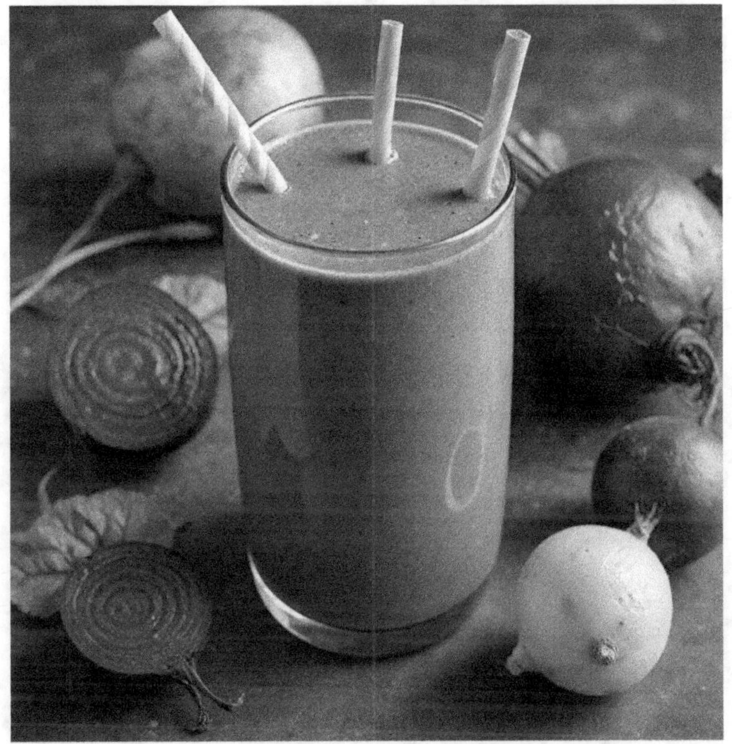

Ingredients for Roasted Beet and Ginger Smoothie:

- 1 medium beet, roasted and peeled
- 1/2 inch piece of fresh ginger, peeled

- 1 small apple, cored and chopped
- 1/2 cup unsweetened almond milk
- 1/2 cup water
- Juice of 1/2 lemon
- 1 tablespoon chia seeds

Instructions:

1. Begin by preheating your oven to 400°F (200°C). Wrap the beet in aluminum foil and roast in the oven for about 45-50 minutes or until tender. Allow it to cool, then peel.

2. Place the roasted beet, fresh ginger, and chopped apple into a blender. Add unsweetened almond milk and water for liquid. This will help in blending and give a smooth consistency.

3. Add the lemon juice and chia seeds. Lemon juice not only enhances flavor but also adds a good dose of vitamin C, while chia seeds provide omega-3 fatty acids and additional fiber.

4. Blend all the ingredients until smooth. If the smoothie is too thick, you can add a bit more water or almond milk to reach your preferred consistency.

5. Taste and adjust the flavors as necessary, adding more lemon juice or ginger according to your preference.

Nutritional Information:

- Calories: 180
- Carbohydrates: 32g
- Fiber: 8g

- Protein: 4g
- Fat: 4g

Serving Size:

This recipe yields approximately 2 servings. Each serving is about
1 cup.

Cooking Time

The total time including preparation and cooking is about 60
minutes, primarily due to the beet roasting process.

Sweet Potato and Cinnamon Smoothie

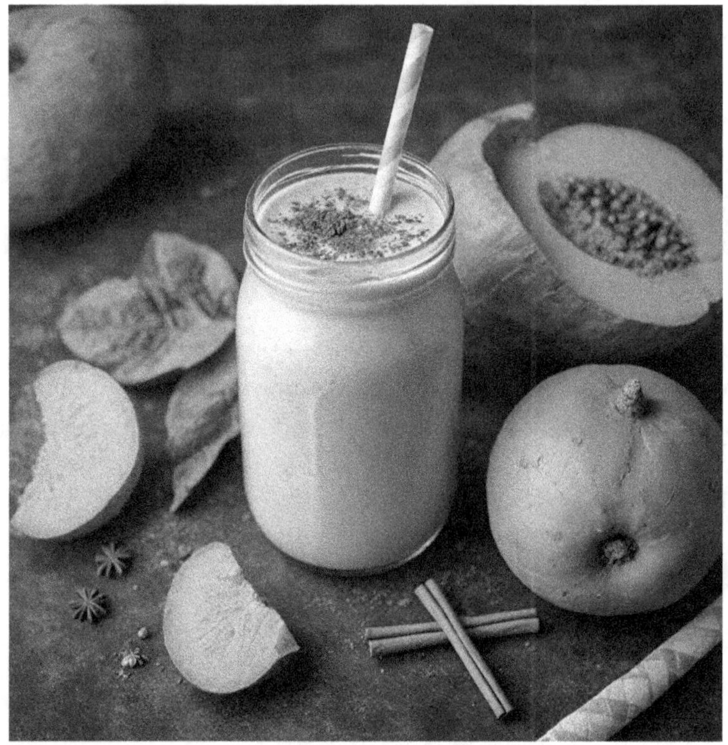

Ingredients:

- 1 medium sweet potato, cooked and peeled

- 1/2 teaspoon ground cinnamon

- 1 cup unsweetened almond milk

- 1 tablespoon almond butter

- 1/2 banana, preferably frozen

- A pinch of sea salt

- Ice cubes (optional, for a thicker smoothie)

Instructions:

1. Start by ensuring your sweet potato is cooked thoroughly and cooled. You can bake, steam, or microwave the sweet potato until tender.

2. Place the cooked sweet potato in a blender along with the cinnamon, unsweetened almond milk, almond butter, and banana.

3. Add a pinch of sea salt to enhance the flavors, adjusting according to your taste preferences.

4. Blend on high until the mixture becomes smooth. If the smoothie is too thick for your liking, you can add more almond milk to adjust the consistency.

5. If a colder or thicker consistency is desired, add ice cubes and blend again until smooth.

6. Pour into a glass and enjoy immediately.

Nutritional Information:

- Calories: Approximately 290 per serving
- Carbohydrates: 44g
- Dietary Fiber: 6g
- Sugars: 18g
- Protein: 6g
- Fat: 10g

Serving Size: This recipe yields about 1-2 servings, depending on your meal planning needs.

Cooking Time: Preparation time is about 5 minutes, assuming the sweet potato is already cooked. If you need to cook the sweet potato, this can add about 30-45 minutes, depending on the cooking method used.

Cauliflower and Berry Smoothie

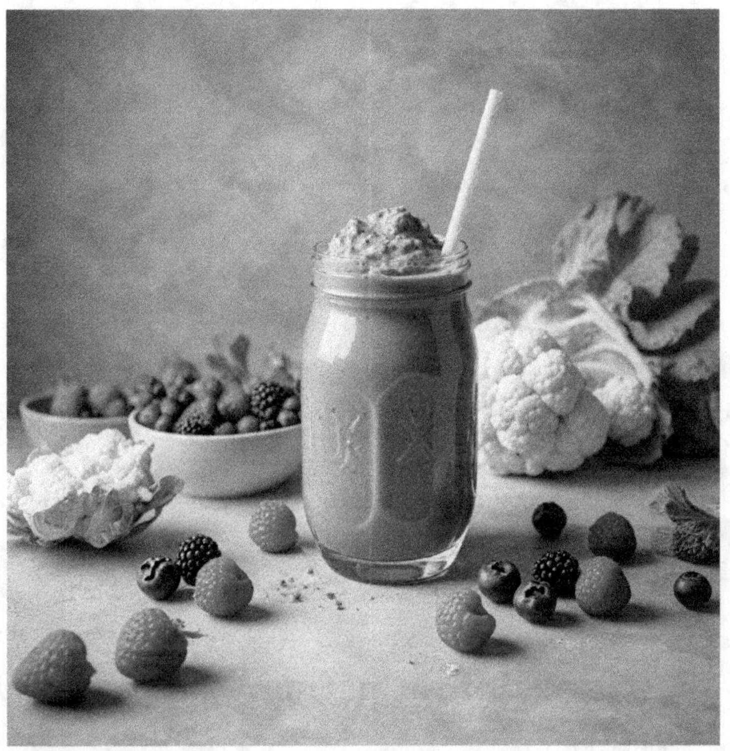

Ingredients:

- 1/2 cup chopped raw cauliflower
- 1/2 cup frozen mixed berries (such as blueberries, strawberries, and blackberries)
- 1 cup unsweetened almond milk
- 1 tablespoon chia seeds
- 1/2 teaspoon vanilla extract

- Ice cubes (optional, for a thicker smoothie)

Instructions:

1. Begin by preparing the cauliflower, ensuring it is washed and chopped into small pieces. This allows for smoother blending and a creamier texture in the smoothie.
2. Place the chopped cauliflower, frozen berries, almond milk, chia seeds, and vanilla extract into a blender.
3. Blend on high until the mixture is completely smooth. If the smoothie is too thick, add a little more almond milk to adjust the consistency. If you prefer a thicker smoothie, add a few ice cubes and blend again.
4. Taste and adjust the sweetness if necessary. For a diabetic-friendly option, avoid sugar and opt for a small amount of stevia or monk fruit sweetener if more sweetness is desired.

Nutritional Information:

- Calories: 150
- Carbohydrates: 18g
- Fiber: 5g
- Protein: 4g
- Fat: 7g
- Sugars: 10g (natural sugars from the berries)

Serving Size:

- This recipe yields one serving, making it easy to control portion size and nutritional intake.

Cooking Time:
- Prep time: 5 minutes
- Blend time: 2 minutes
- Total time: 7 minutes

Asparagus and Lemon Smoothie

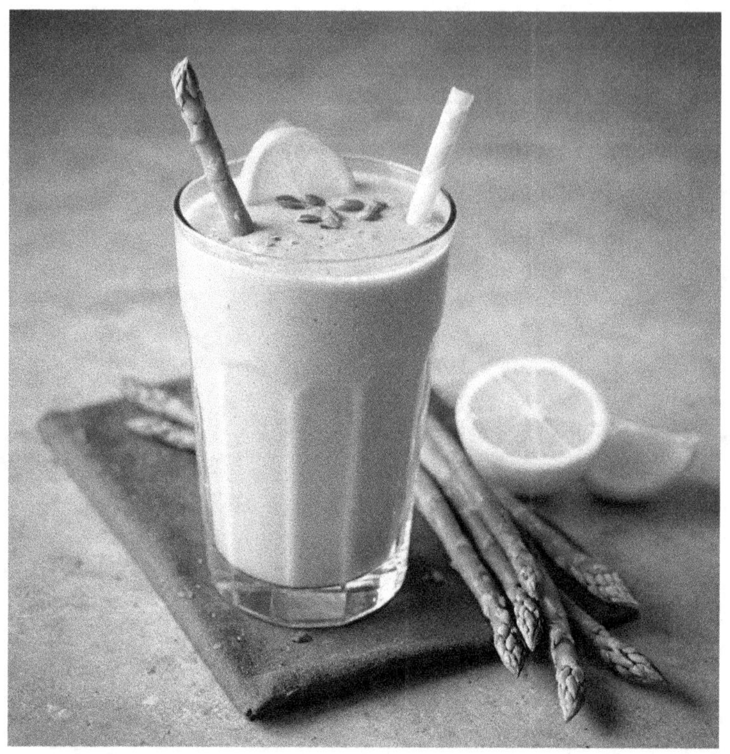

Ingredients

- 1 cup chopped asparagus, tips and mid-sections only (tough ends removed)
- Juice of 1 lemon
- 1/2 avocado
- 1 cup unsweetened almond milk

- 1 tablespoon flaxseeds
- 1/2 teaspoon grated ginger
- Ice cubes (optional, for a chilled smoothie)

Instructions

1. Wash the asparagus thoroughly and chop into manageable pieces, discarding the tough ends.
2. Place the chopped asparagus, lemon juice, avocado, almond milk, flaxseeds, and ginger into a blender.
3. Blend on high until the mixture becomes smooth and creamy. If the smoothie is too thick, add more almond milk to reach the desired consistency.
4. If a chilled smoothie is preferred, add a handful of ice cubes and blend again until smooth.
5. Taste and adjust the flavors as needed, adding more lemon juice or ginger for extra zing.

Nutritional Information:

- Calories: 190
- Total Fat: 12 g
- Saturated Fat: 2 g
- Cholesterol: 0 mg
- Sodium: 70 mg
- Total Carbohydrates: 18 g
- Dietary Fiber: 8 g
- Sugars: 5 g

- Protein: 4 g

Serving Size: This recipe yields approximately 2 servings.

Cooking Time: The total time required to prepare and blend this smoothie is about 10 minutes.

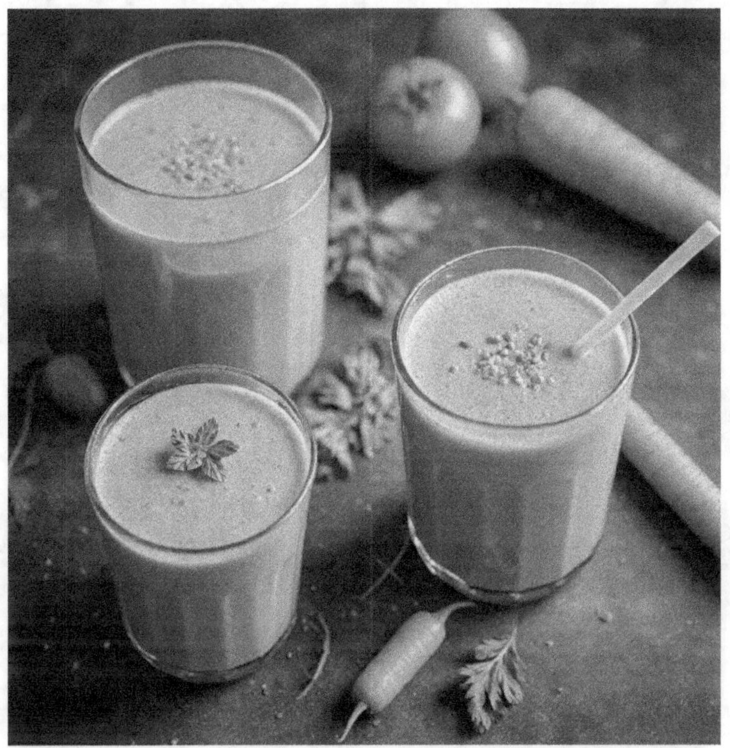

Ingredients for Spicy Tomato and Carrot Smoothie:

- 2 large tomatoes, chopped
- 1 large carrot, peeled and chopped
- 1 small red bell pepper, deseeded and chopped
- 1/2 cucumber, peeled and chopped
- 1/2 tsp of fresh ginger, grated

- 1/4 tsp of cayenne pepper (adjust according to taste)
- 1 tbsp of lemon juice
- 1/2 cup of cold water or vegetable broth
- Salt to taste
- A handful of ice cubes

Instructions:

1. Start by preparing all the vegetables – wash, chop, and measure them as listed.
2. Place the tomatoes, carrot, bell pepper, and cucumber into the blender.
3. Add the grated ginger, cayenne pepper, and lemon juice to the mix. These ingredients will give the smoothie a nice zest and spice.
4. Pour in the cold water or vegetable broth, which helps in blending the ingredients smoothly and adds an extra layer of flavor.
5. Blend on high until all the ingredients are thoroughly combined and the mixture is smooth.
6. Taste and adjust the seasoning with salt, and add ice cubes before giving it one last blend to chill the smoothie.
7. Serve immediately.

Nutritional Information:

- Calories: Approximately 120 per serving
- Carbohydrates: 18g
- Dietary Fiber: 5g

- Sugars: 12g
- Protein: 3g
- Fat: 1g

Serving Size:

- This recipe yields about 2 servings.

Cooking Time:

- Total preparation and blending time is approximately 10 minutes.

Butternut Squash and Turmeric Smoothie

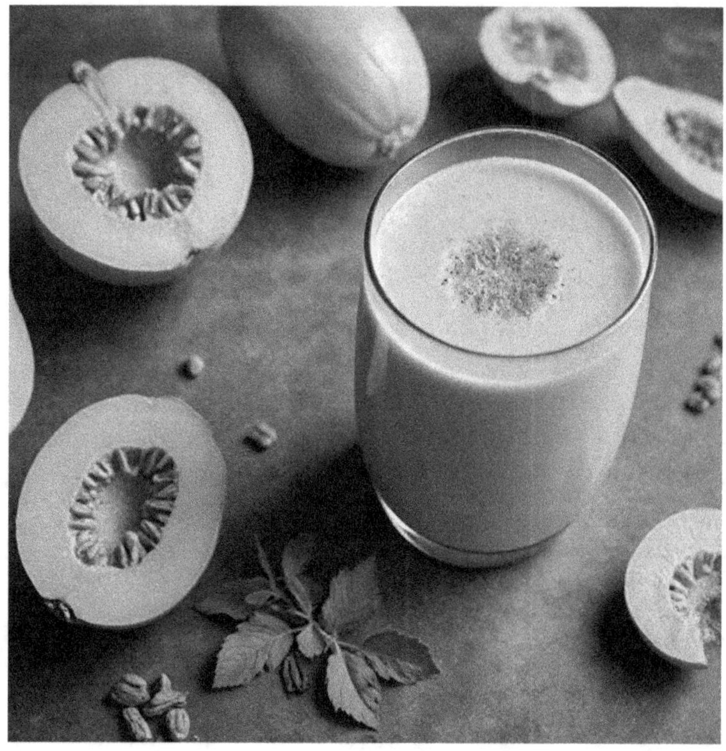

Ingredients:

- 1 cup roasted butternut squash, cooled
- 1/2 banana, preferably slightly underripe
- 1 cup unsweetened almond milk
- 1/2 teaspoon ground turmeric
- 1/4 teaspoon ground cinnamon

- 1 tablespoon chia seeds
- 1 scoop unflavored or vanilla protein powder (optional for added protein)
- Ice cubes (adjust quantity for desired thickness)

Instructions:

1. Start by preparing the butternut squash. Peel, seed, and cut the squash into cubes, then roast in an oven at 400 degrees Fahrenheit for about 30 minutes or until soft and slightly caramelized. Allow it to cool.
2. Place the cooled butternut squash cubes into a blender. Add the half banana, almond milk, turmeric, cinnamon, and chia seeds. If using, add the protein powder.
3. Blend on high until the mixture reaches a smooth and creamy consistency. Add ice cubes and blend again until the smoothie reaches your preferred thickness.
4. Taste and adjust the seasoning, perhaps adding a bit more cinnamon or a touch of vanilla extract for extra flavor.

Nutritional Information:

Each serving of this smoothie offers a balanced mix of nutrients conducive to a diabetic diet. Approximately:
- Calories: 200
- Carbohydrates: 35 g
- Fiber: 7 g
- Protein: 8 g

- Fat: 4 g
- Sugars: 12 g (from natural sources)
The nutritional values can vary slightly based on the brand of
protein powder used, if any.

Serving Size:

This recipe yields about 2 cups, suitable for one large serving or
two smaller servings if preferred as a light dinner supplement.

Cooking Time:

Preparation time is around 45 minutes, including the 30 minutes
needed to roast the butternut squash. The actual blending takes
no more than 5 minutes.

Eggplant and Red Berry Smoothie

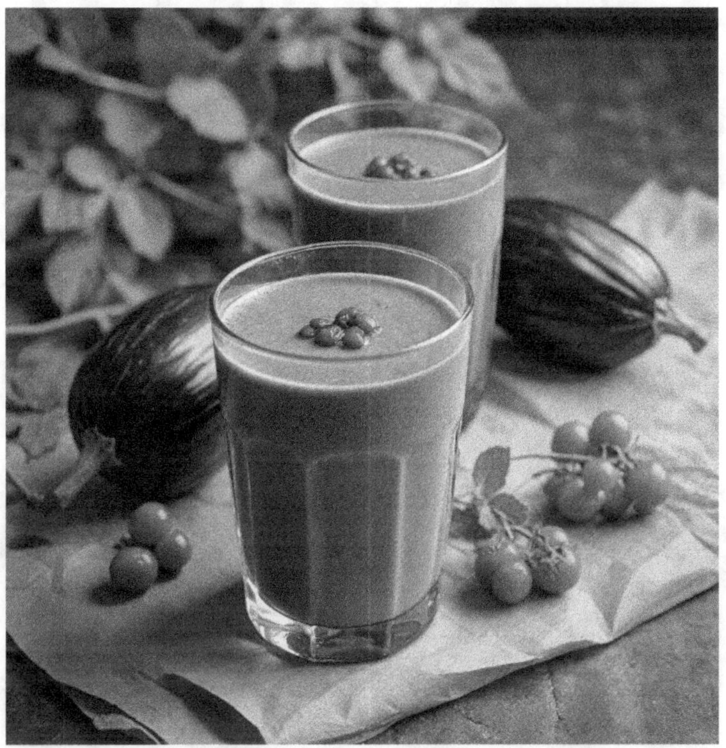

Ingredient List:

- 1/2 medium eggplant, peeled and diced
- 1 cup mixed red berries (like strawberries and raspberries), fresh or frozen
- 1/2 cup unsweetened almond milk
- 1/4 cup Greek yogurt, plain
- 1 tablespoon flaxseeds

- 1 teaspoon vanilla extract
- Ice cubes (optional, adjust based on desired thickness)

Instructions:

1. Begin by steaming the diced eggplant until it is tender, about 6-8 minutes. Allow it to cool slightly.
2. In a blender, combine the steamed eggplant, red berries, almond milk, Greek yogurt, flaxseeds, and vanilla extract. If using ice, add it at this time.
3. Blend on high speed until the mixture is smooth and creamy. If the smoothie is too thick, add a little more almond milk to reach the desired consistency.
4. Taste and adjust the sweetness if necessary; depending on your dietary needs and preferences, you might add a touch of a diabetic-friendly sweetener.
5. Serve immediately for the best flavor and texture.

Nutritional Information:

- Calories: Approximately 200 per serving
- Carbohydrates: 28 grams
- Fiber: 7 grams
- Protein: 8 grams
- Fat: 6 grams

Serving Size:

- This recipe yields about 2 servings.

Cooking Time:

- Preparation time: 10 minutes
- Cooking time: 8 minutes
- Total time: 18 minutes

Creamy Avocado and Cacao Smoothie

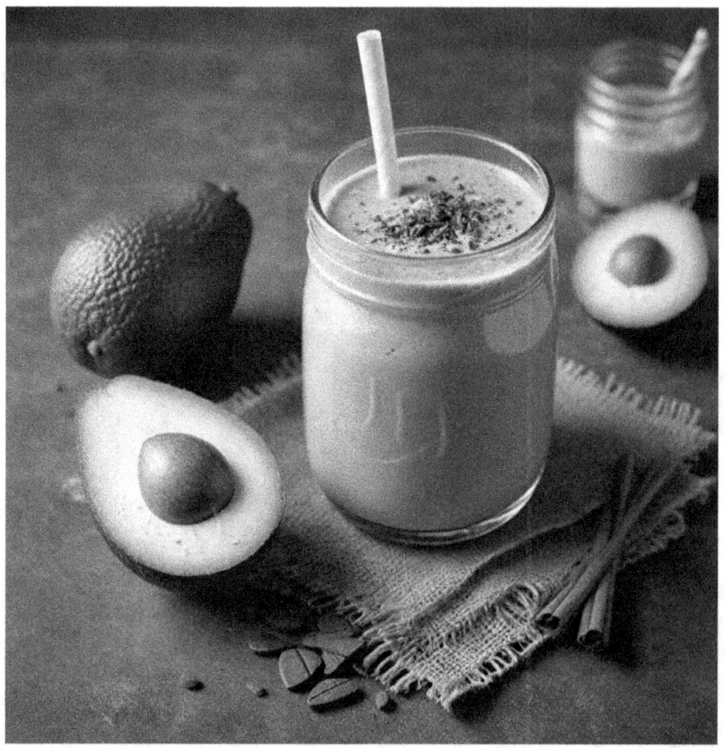

Ingredients:

- 1 ripe avocado, peeled and pitted
- 2 tablespoons raw cacao powder
- 1 cup unsweetened almond milk
- 1/2 teaspoon vanilla extract
- 1 tablespoon chia seeds
- 2 teaspoons erythritol or another low-calorie sweetener

- Ice cubes (optional, for thicker consistency)

Instructions:

1. Start by adding the almond milk to your blender to create a fluid base.
2. Add the peeled and pitted avocado and raw cacao powder.
3. Incorporate the vanilla extract, chia seeds, and sweetener.
4. Blend on high until the mixture is completely smooth. If a thicker consistency is desired, add ice cubes and blend again.
5. Taste and adjust the sweetness if necessary.

Nutritional Information:

- Calories: 345
- Total Fat: 24g
- Saturated Fat: 4g
- Carbohydrates: 27g
- Fiber: 12g
- Sugars: 2g
- Protein: 6g

Serving Size:

- Makes 1 large serving or 2 smaller servings.

Cooking Time:

- Prep time: 5 minutes

- Blend time: 2 minutes

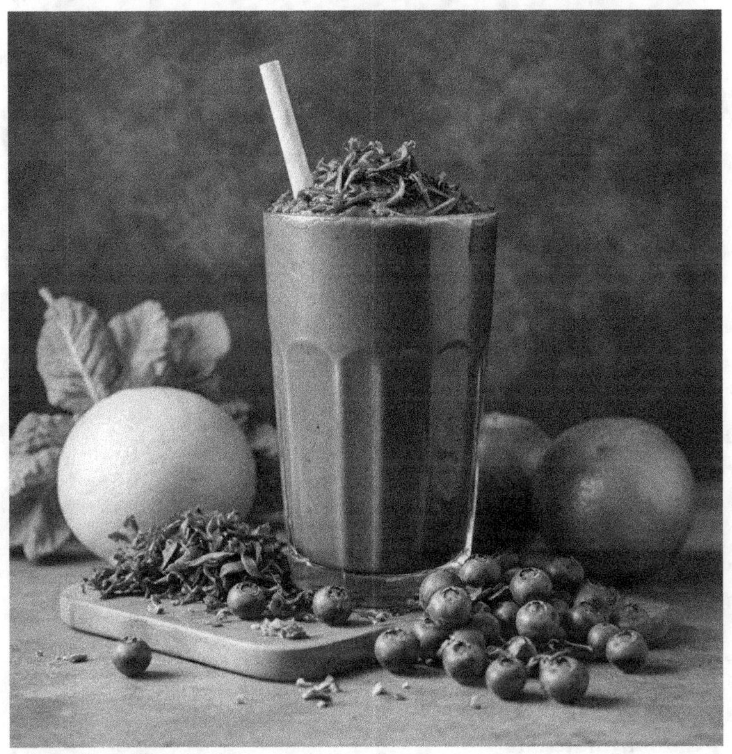

Ingredients:

- 1 cup red cabbage, chopped
- 1/2 cup blueberries, fresh or frozen
- 1 small banana
- 1 tablespoon chia seeds
- 1/2 cup unsweetened almond milk
- 1/2 cup water

- Ice cubes (optional, for a colder smoothie)

Instructions:

1. Start by placing the almond milk and water in the blender to create a liquid base.
2. Add the chopped red cabbage, blueberries, and banana to the blender. If using frozen blueberries, they can also help chill the smoothie, potentially eliminating the need for ice.
3. Sprinkle the chia seeds into the blender.
4. Blend on high until all components are thoroughly combined and the smoothie achieves a creamy, smooth consistency.
5. If the smoothie is too thick, add a little more water or almond milk to adjust the consistency.
6. Serve immediately for the best taste and nutrient retention.

Nutritional Information:

- Calories: 210
- Carbohydrates: 44g
- Fiber: 8g
- Protein: 4g
- Fat: 4g
- Sugar: 18g (natural sugars from the fruits)

Serving Size:

This recipe yields approximately 1 large serving or can be divided into 2 smaller servings if preferred.

Cooking Time:

The total preparation and blending time for this smoothie is about 5 minutes, making it an excellent option for a quick and easy dinner.

Kale and Green Apple Smoothie

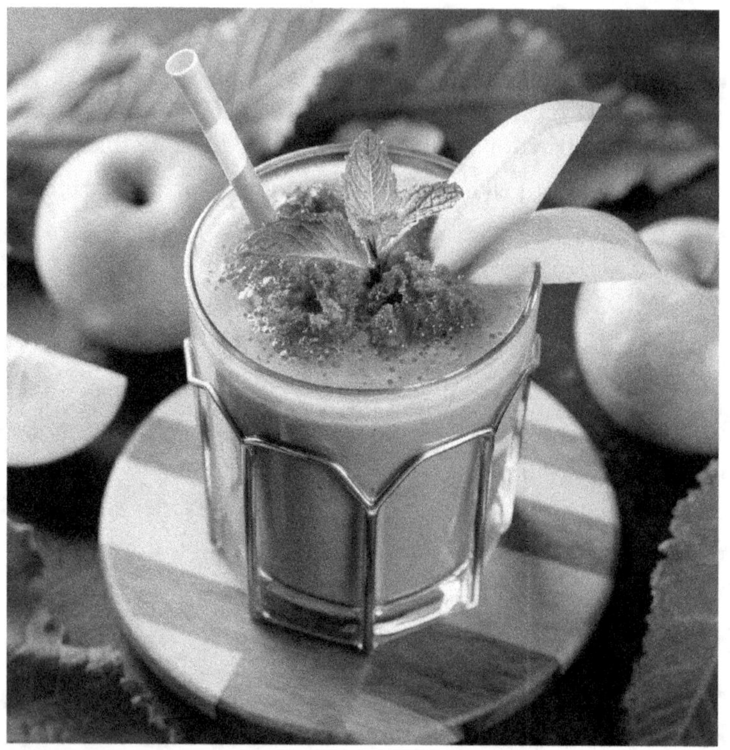

Ingredients:

- 1 cup chopped kale, stems removed
- 1 green apple, cored and sliced
- 1/2 cup unsweetened Greek yogurt
- 1 tablespoon flaxseeds
- 1/2 cup almond milk
- 1/2 teaspoon cinnamon

- Ice cubes (optional)

Instructions:

1. Place the kale and almond milk in the blender first. Blend on high until the kale is finely chopped.
2. Add the green apple, Greek yogurt, flaxseeds, and cinnamon to the blender.
3. If a colder consistency is desired, add ice cubes.
4. Blend on high until smooth and creamy. Ensure all components are fully incorporated, and the texture is to your liking.

Nutritional Information:

- Calories: 190
- Carbohydrates: 27g
- Fiber: 5g
- Protein: 10g
- Fat: 6g
- Sugar: 15g

Serving Size:

- Makes 1 serving (approximately 16 ounces)

Cooking Time:

- Prep and blend time: Approximately 5 minutes

Chapter: 5 Snack and Dessert Smoothies

Almond and Date Smoothie

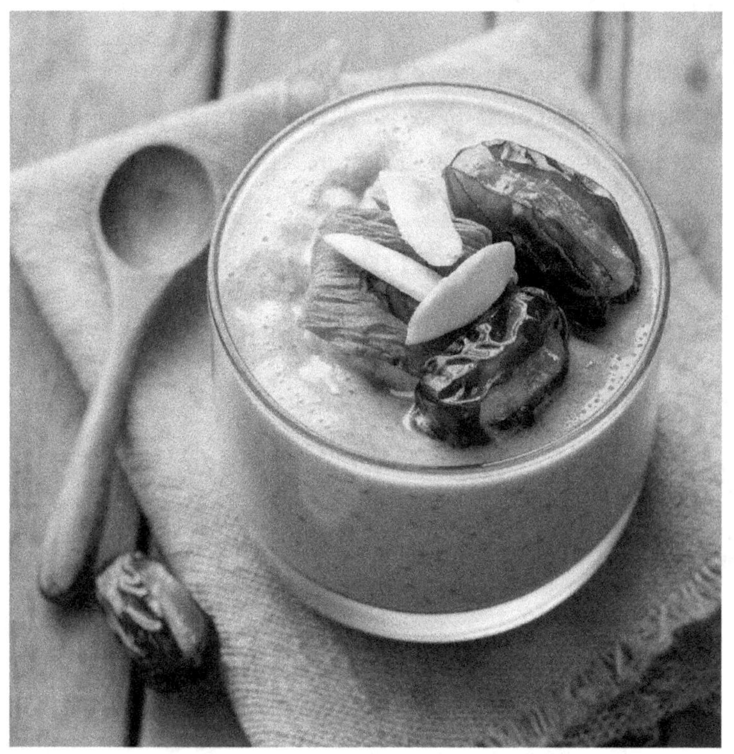

Ingredients for Almond and Date Smoothie:

- 1/4 cup whole almonds, soaked overnight and drained
- 2 Medjool dates, pitted
- 1 cup unsweetened almond milk
- 1/2 teaspoon ground cinnamon
- 1 small frozen banana
- Ice cubes (optional, for a thicker smoothie)

Instructions:

1. Place the soaked and drained almonds, pitted dates, and almond milk into a blender. Blend on high speed until the mixture is smooth and the nuts are finely ground.
2. Add the frozen banana, cinnamon, and ice cubes if using. Continue to blend until the smoothie reaches your desired consistency.
3. Pour the smoothie into a glass and garnish with a sprinkle of cinnamon or a few almond slivers if desired.

Nutritional Information:

- Calories: 320
- Total Fat: 15g
- Saturated Fat: 1g
- Total Carbohydrates: 44g
- Dietary Fiber: 7g
- Sugars: 32g
- Protein: 8g

Serving Size:

This recipe yields approximately one serving, making it a perfect single snack or dessert portion.

Cooking Time:

The total preparation and blending time is about 10 minutes, assuming that the almonds have been pre-soaked.

Raspberry Lime Smoothie

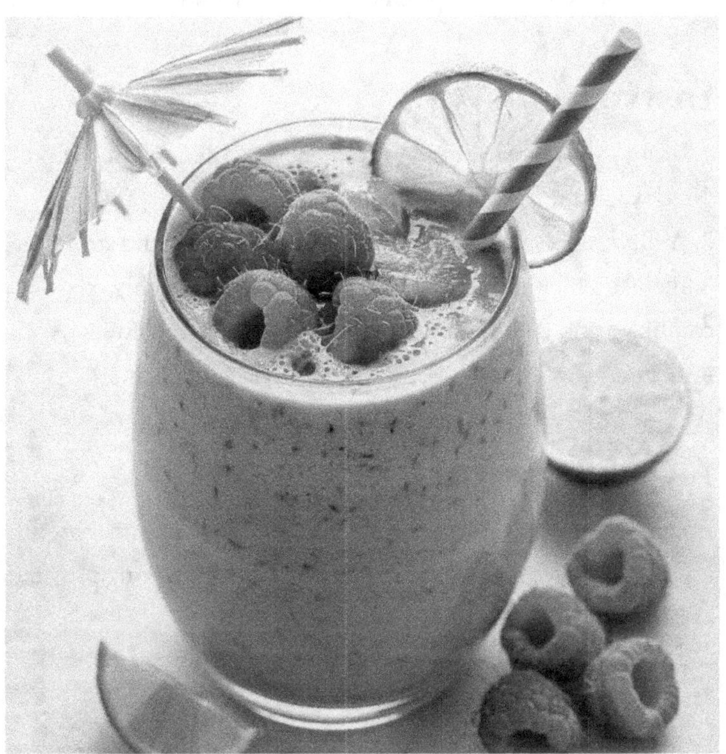

To prepare this smoothie, you will need the following ingredients:

- 1 cup fresh or frozen raspberries
- Juice of 1 lime
- 1/2 cup unsweetened almond milk
- 1/2 cup Greek yogurt, plain and unsweetened
- 1 tablespoon chia seeds

- Ice cubes (optional, for a thicker consistency)
- A few drops of stevia (optional, for added sweetness)

Instructions:

1. Begin by placing the raspberries, lime juice, almond milk, and Greek yogurt into your blender.
2. Add the chia seeds, and if you're using, ice cubes and stevia.
3. Blend on high until all the ingredients are thoroughly combined and the mixture achieves your desired consistency.
4. Taste and adjust the sweetness with stevia if needed.

Nutritional Information:

Each serving of this smoothie offers a balanced nutritional profile ideal for diabetes management. Here's what each serving provides:
- Calories: 190
- Protein: 9 grams
- Fat: 5 grams
- Carbohydrates: 28 grams
- Fiber: 8 grams
- Sugars: 12 grams (natural sugars from the raspberries and lime)

Serving Size:

This recipe yields approximately 2 servings.

Cooking Time:

The total preparation time for the Raspberry Lime Smoothie is about 5 minutes, making it a quick and easy option for a snack or dessert.

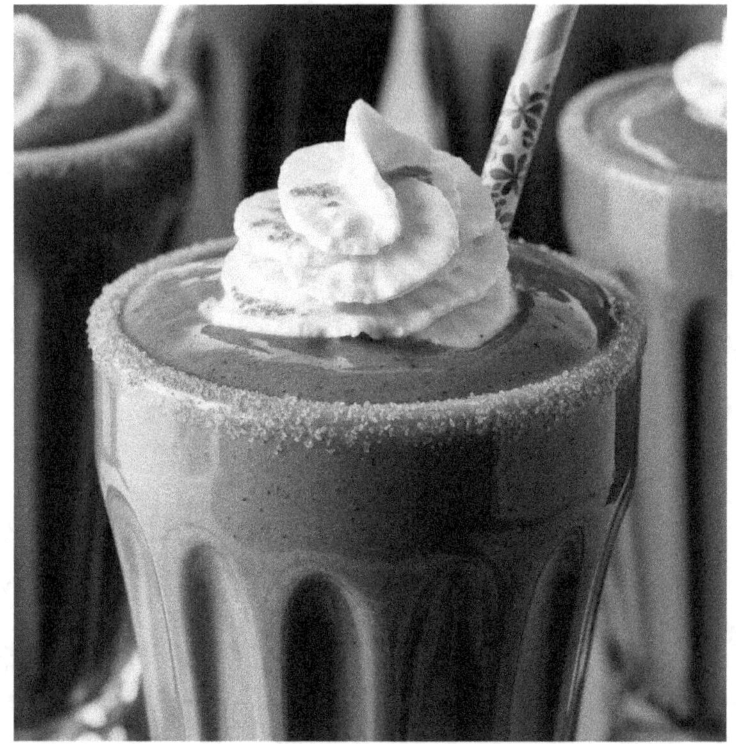

Ingredient List for Cacao and Banana Smoothie:

- 1 ripe banana, preferably frozen
- 1 tablespoon unsweetened cacao powder
- 1/2 cup unsweetened almond milk
- 1/4 teaspoon ground cinnamon
- 1 tablespoon chia seeds

- A few ice cubes
- Optional sweetener: stevia or a sugar substitute to taste

Instructions:

1. Place the banana, cacao powder, almond milk, ground cinnamon, and chia seeds in the blender.
2. Add ice cubes to the mixture.
3. Blend on high speed until the mixture is smooth and creamy. If the smoothie is too thick, you can add a bit more almond milk to reach the desired consistency.
4. Taste and add a sweetener if necessary, blending again briefly to mix through.

Nutritional Information:

- Calories: Approximately 200
- Carbohydrates: 30g
- Dietary Fiber: 7g
- Sugars: 12g (natural sugars from the banana)
- Protein: 5g
- Fat: 6g (primarily healthy fats from chia seeds)

Serving Size:

- This recipe makes one serving, ideal for one person as a snack or dessert alternative.

Cooking Time:

- Total preparation and blending time is about 5 minutes.

Pear Ginger Smoothie

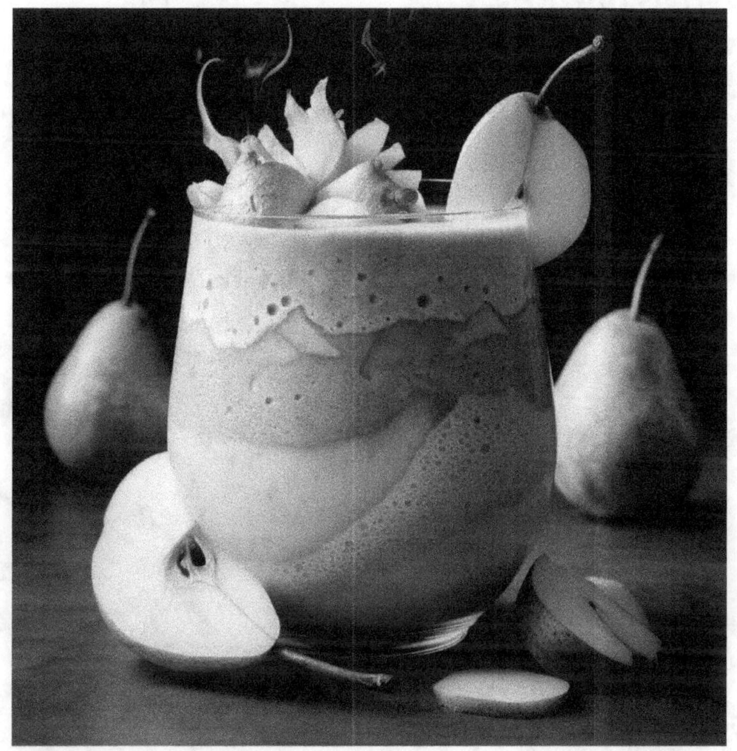

Ingredients:

- 1 ripe pear, cored and chopped
- 1/2 teaspoon fresh ginger, grated
- 1 tablespoon chia seeds
- 1/2 cup unsweetened almond milk
- 1/2 cup Greek yogurt, plain
- A handful of ice cubes

Instructions:

1. Place the chopped pear and grated ginger in the blender.
2. Add the chia seeds for a fiber boost, which can help manage blood sugar levels.
3. Pour in the unsweetened almond milk and Greek yogurt for a creamy texture and a dose of protein.
4. Add a handful of ice cubes to chill and thicken the smoothie.
5. Blend on high until the mixture is smooth and creamy. Ensure all ingredients are thoroughly combined and the smoothie reaches your preferred consistency.

Nutritional Information:

- Calories: 210
- Carbohydrates: 35g
- Fiber: 7g
- Sugars: 20g
- Protein: 13g
- Fat: 3g

Serving Size:

This recipe yields approximately one serving of 16 ounces, making it an ideal size for a fulfilling snack or a light dessert.

Cooking Time:

The total preparation and blending time is around 5 minutes, making this smoothie a quick and easy option for those busy days or when you need a quick dessert fix.

Walnut and Fig Smoothie

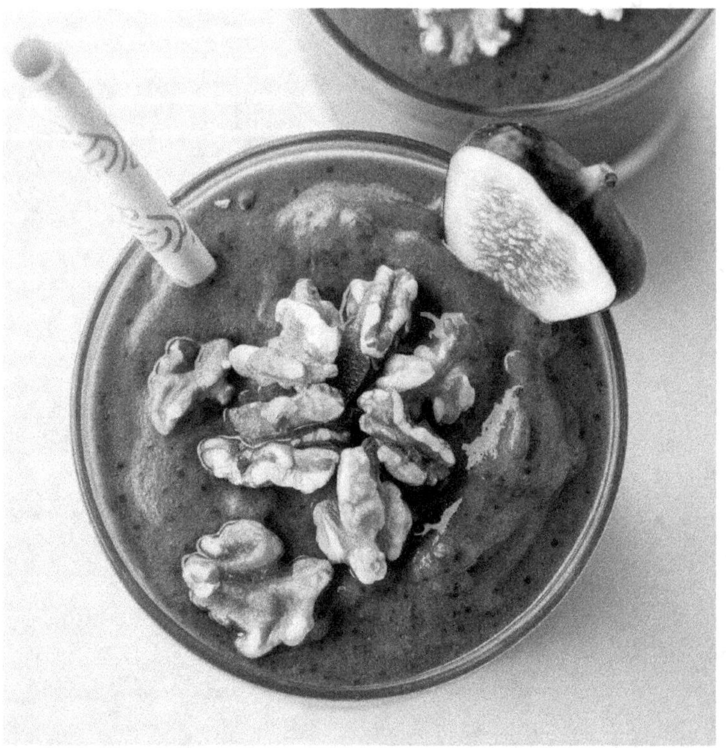

Ingredients:

- 3 dried figs, stems removed
- 1/4 cup raw walnuts
- 1 cup unsweetened almond milk
- 1/2 teaspoon ground cinnamon
- 1/2 frozen banana, sliced
- Ice cubes, as needed for thickness

Instructions:

1. Place the figs in a small bowl with warm water. Let them soak for about 10 minutes to soften.

2. In a blender, combine the soaked figs (minus the soaking water), walnuts, almond milk, cinnamon, and frozen banana.

3. Add ice cubes according to the desired thickness and blend until smooth. For a thinner smoothie, add more almond milk.

Nutritional Information (per serving):

- Calories: 290
- Carbohydrates: 38 g
- Fiber: 6 g
- Protein: 6 g
- Fat: 15 g
- Sugar: 20 g (natural sugars from the figs and banana)

Serving Size:

- Makes 1 serving (approximately 12 ounces)

Cooking Time:

- Total preparation time: 15 minutes (including the time for soaking the figs)

Chapter: 6 Specialty Smoothies

Detox and Cleanse Smoothies

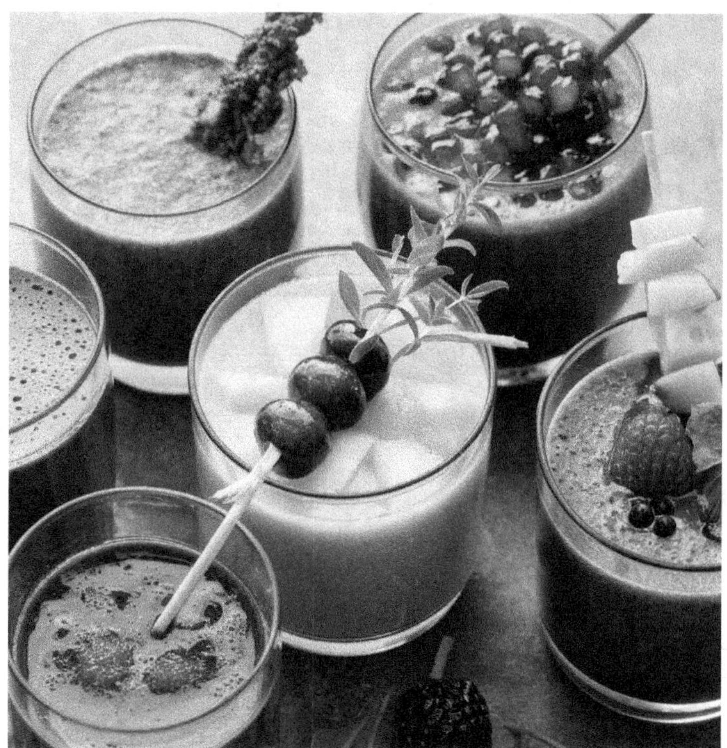

Ingredients:

- 1 cup fresh spinach
- 1/2 cucumber, peeled and sliced
- 1 green apple, cored and chopped (skin on)
- 1/2 avocado

- 1 tablespoon chia seeds

- 1 cup unsweetened almond milk

- Juice of 1/2 lemon

- A few mint leaves for extra freshness

Instructions:

1. Begin by washing all the fresh produce thoroughly.

2. Place spinach, cucumber, green apple, and avocado into the blender.

3. Add chia seeds and mint leaves.

4. Pour in the unsweetened almond milk and squeeze in the lemon juice.

5. Blend on high until smooth. If the smoothie is too thick, you can add a little more almond milk to reach the desired consistency.

Nutritional Information:

- Calories: 220
- Carbohydrates: 24 g
- Fiber: 9 g
- Protein: 4 g
- Fat: 12 g
- Sugar: 12 g

Serving Size: Makes about 16 ounces (2 servings)

Cooking Time: Prep and blend time approximately 5 minutes

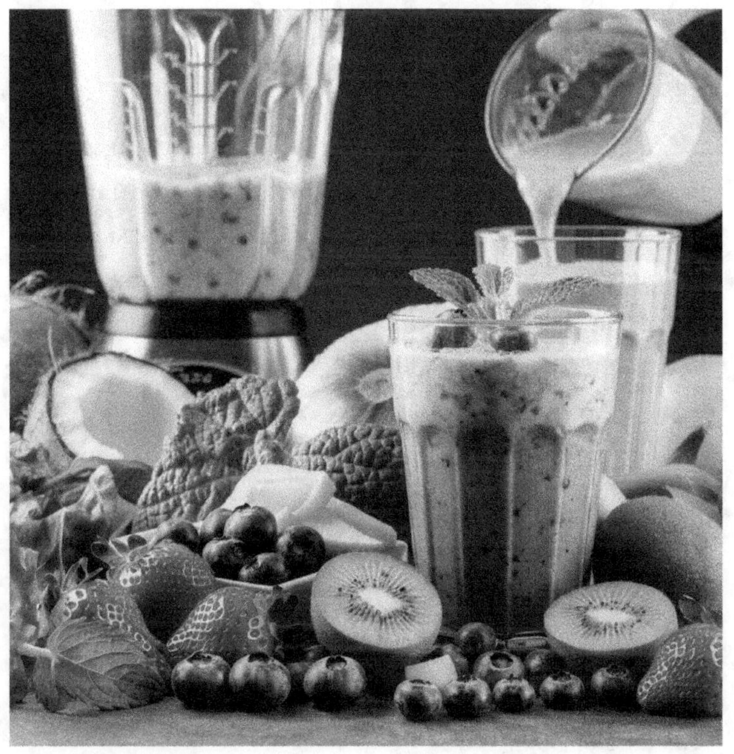

Ingredients:

- 1 cup fresh spinach
- 1 small cucumber, chopped
- 1/2 green apple, cored and sliced
- 1/4 avocado
- 1 tablespoon chia seeds
- 1 cup unsweetened almond milk

- 1 scoop vanilla protein powder
- Ice cubes (optional)

Instructions:

1. Place the spinach, cucumber, and green apple in the blender first, adding the avocado, chia seeds, and protein powder on top.
2. Pour in the almond milk and add ice if desired for a colder smoothie.
3. Blend on high until all components are completely smooth. If the smoothie is too thick, add a little more almond milk to achieve the desired consistency.
4. Serve immediately for the best flavor and nutrient retention.

Nutritional Information:

- Calories: 235
- Total Fat: 8g
- Saturated Fat: 1g
- Cholesterol: 30mg
- Sodium: 125mg
- Total Carbohydrates: 21g
- Dietary Fiber: 8g
- Sugars: 10g
- Protein: 20g

Serving Size:

- Makes 1 serving (approximately 16 ounces)

Cooking Time:

- Preparation time: 10 minutes
- No cooking required

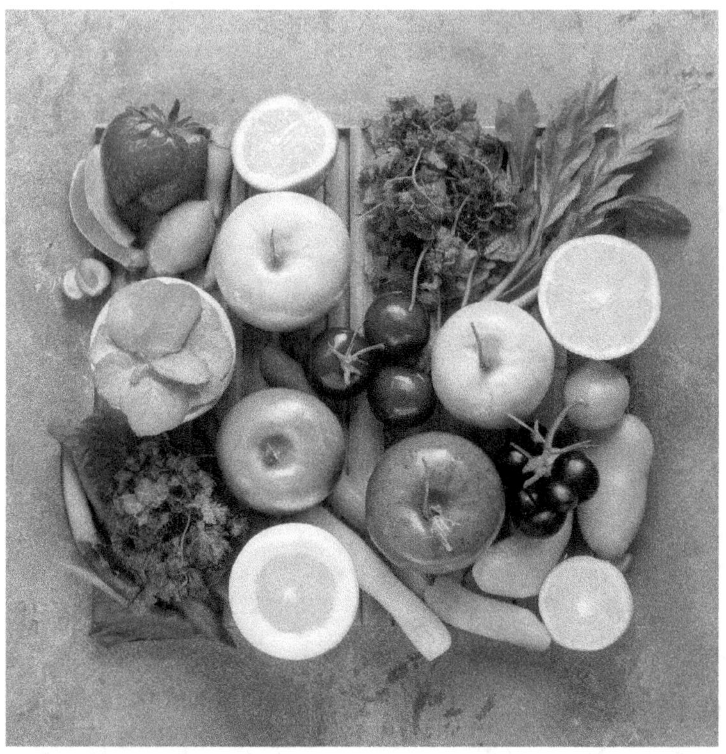

Ingredients:

- 1 cup unsweetened almond milk

- 1/2 cup blueberries (fresh or frozen)

- 1 tablespoon chia seeds

- 1/2 teaspoon ground cinnamon

- 1 scoop protein powder (vanilla or unflavored)

- Ice cubes (optional, adjust according to desired thickness)

Instructions:

1. Place all ingredients in the blender, starting with the almond milk to facilitate smoother blending.

2. Add the blueberries, chia seeds, and ground cinnamon on top of the liquid.

3. Add the scoop of protein powder last to prevent it from sticking to the bottom.

4. Blend on high until the mixture is smooth and creamy. If using ice cubes, add them last and blend until the desired consistency is achieved.

Nutritional Information:

- Calories: 180
- Carbohydrates: 18 g
- Fiber: 5 g
- Protein: 15 g
- Fat: 7 g
- Sugars: 7 g

Serving Size:

- Makes 1 serving (approximately 16 oz)

Preparation Time:

- Total time: 5 minutes

Conclusion

The "Diabetic Smoothie Cookbook 2024" concludes with a thoughtful reflection on the transformative power of integrating smoothies into a diabetic diet. The book emphasizes that smoothies are more than just a convenient and delicious way to consume a variety of essential nutrients; they are a vital tool for managing diabetes effectively and enjoying a higher quality of life.

Through its carefully curated recipes, the cookbook demonstrates that managing blood sugar levels does not mean sacrificing flavor or the joy of eating. Each recipe is crafted to provide a balanced blend of nutrients that support blood sugar control, including fibers, proteins, and healthy fats, all of which are crucial for minimizing glycemic spikes. This approach allows individuals living with diabetes to indulge in a diverse array of flavors and textures without fear of destabilizing their glucose levels.

Furthermore, the book reinforces the importance of understanding the components of each smoothie. By educating readers on the nutritional impact of ingredients, the cookbook empowers them with the knowledge to make informed choices about their diet beyond just the pages of the book. This education is intended to serve as a foundation for a sustainable lifestyle change, encouraging readers to embrace smoothies as a part of a holistic approach to diabetes management.

The conclusion also highlights the flexibility offered by the recipes within the book. Readers are encouraged to experiment with substituting ingredients and adjusting proportions to cater to their personal preferences and nutritional needs. This adaptability ensures that the smoothies can be integrated seamlessly into any diabetic diet, making it easier for individuals to maintain consistent blood sugar levels while enjoying diverse and satisfying meals.

In closing, the cookbook calls on readers to view these smoothies as a daily ritual, a moment of pleasure that nourishes both the body and the soul. It invites them to share their creations and experiences with others, fostering a community of support among those managing diabetes. By exchanging stories and tips, readers can find encouragement and inspiration, reinforcing the idea that a diabetes diagnosis can be the start of a rich, vibrant culinary adventure—not a restriction.

Ultimately, the "Diabetic Smoothie Cookbook 2024" concludes on a note of optimism, underscoring the possibility of living a full and active life with diabetes. It assures readers that with the right tools, knowledge, and a dash of creativity, they can take control of their health and find joy in every sip. This powerful message serves as a reminder of the cookbook's role not just as a collection of recipes, but as a companion in the journey towards wellness and diabetes management.

9 798327 702608